P9-DCP-422

Praise for *A Mother's Final Gift*:

"This book is moving, uplifting, and ennobling. While the topic is a daunting one, it's handled with such sensitivity and insight – and, yes, love – that you are forced to reexamine your fears about death and dying... and dispense with them."
– John Gray, Executive Producer, Creator, Director: CBS-TV "The Ghost Whisperer"

"A rare and touching account! If you would like to deepen your connection with your family, especially during the time of a passing of a loved one, this book will give you courage, inspiration, and a higher vision that will soothe your soul and help you navigate transition. It's a magnificent testament to love and the power of family to navigate transition."
– Alan Cohen, author of Linden's Last Life.

"The Vissell family has written a beautiful and moving account of their mother's (and grandmother's) death. Despite her challenges, Louise Wollenberg lived her dying as a celebration of life. Her open and courageous heart became a portal to the other side, and her presence became a place of healing. This book will comfort and inspire."
– Michael Kearney, MD, FRCPI, Medical Director of the Palliative Care Service at Santa Barbara Cottage Hospital and Associate Medical Director at Visiting Nurse and Hospice Care.

"This is a goose bump book, a 10 hankie page-turner and a real primer for a loving, dying experience. Anyone who is caring for a loved one in the last stages of life or wanting to better understand conscious dying will gain comfort and insight from its pages."
– Caroline Sutherland, author of The Body Knows

"I have sat at many bedsides of people who were dying, and heard many speak of their fear of becoming a burden upon their families. This book strongly speaks to how this perceived 'burden' can be such a huge gift and opportunity, for love, service and growth. A Mother's Final Gift *shows us that our dying isn't just for ourselves, but can be a gift and teaching capable of forever transforming the lives of the people around us. This book is for those who may become caregivers one day, and those who think they might die one day."*
– Bodhi Be, Executive Director, Doorway Into Light.

"Every person connected with the Hospice organization and community will embrace the message of A Mother's Final Gift *and the Vissell family's powerful message of love and hope. I look forward to using and recommending this book as an important resource for staff, volunteers, patients and families."*
– Joan Martin, RN, Hospice Patient Care Administrator

"Honestly portrayed, this end-of-life story is a rich tapestry of insight, courage, love and reconciliation. A Mother's Final Gift *will bring comfort and understanding to families both before and after a loved one's transition. A great addition to the field."*
– Savarna Wiley, Hospice Chaplain

"Much more than a book about death and dying, A Mother's Final Gift *is about living life – and living it to the fullest."*
– Brian Copperstein, Hospice Social Worker

*"*A Mother's Final Gift *is about the many facets of a family's journey toward transformation, and the inspirations they experienced firsthand as they witnessed the great and intimate passage of their beloved mother, grandmother and friend, Louise. As always, the Vissell Family 'live their values' and exemplify to us the meaning of true love."*
– Connection Magazine

"So many people have such a terrible fear of death, and fear not only their own dying process but that of those they care for. Louise met her dying with dignity, without fear, and with a great sense of adventure. What a model this book is for all of us, to have such a conscious and beautiful death, surrounded by those we love, and giving a memorable gift in the process."
– Linda Bloom, LCSW, and Charlie Bloom, MSW, authors of *Secrets of Great Marriages*

"*A Mother's Final Gift is a transparent, intimate and sweetly touching memoir of a mother's death. This is the most powerful and poignant account of a conscious death that we have ever seen, an experience that is deeply bonding for all, overflowing with compassion for our precarious and perishable human condition, and, above all, a joyful celebration of love's omnipresence. This book is an inspiring guide to the adventure of dying and death that is possible for us all.*"
– Rich and Antra Borofsky, Co-directors, Center for the Study of Relationship, Cambridge, MA

A Mother's Final Gift

How One Woman's Courageous Dying Transformed Her Family

By Joyce Vissell, RN, MS
& Barry Vissell, MD
with Rami, Mira,
and John-Nuri Vissell

A Mother's Final Gift:

How One Woman's Courageous Dying Transformed Her Family

Copyright © 2011 by Ramira Publishing
PO Box 2140, Aptos, CA 95001-2140. 800.766.0629 or 831.684.2299.
www.SharedHeart.org.

All rights reserved. No part of this book may be used or reproduced in any manner whatsoever without written permission, except in the case of brief quotations in articles or reviews.

ISBN-13: 978-0-9612720-3-6
Library of Congress Control Number: 2011922141

Printed in the United States of America on acid-free, chlorine-free, and Sustainable Forestry Initiative (SFI) certified paper.

Cover design by Melinda Laughton.
Back cover photo by Sarojani Rohan.

Also by Barry and Joyce Vissell:

The Shared Heart: Relationship Initiations and Celebrations
Models of Love: The Parent-Child Journey
Risk to be Healed: The Heart of Personal and Relationship Growth
Light in the Mirror: A New Way to Understand Relationships
Meant To Be: Miraculous True Stories to Inspire a Lifetime of Love
And by Rami Vissell:
Rami's Book: The Inner Life of a Child

Acknowledgements

We offer our gratitude to Wendy Sherman for being the first person to believe in this project; and to Elsa Dixon for her insightful editing and restructuring of the manuscript.

Thanks to our editors: Leslie Sahler, Ana Fatima Costa, Trish Turpel, Chery Klairwator, Sharon Wesolowski, and Liliana Cartagena

Thank you Melinda Lawton for the beautiful book cover.

Finally, our heart-felt thanks to Hospice of Santa Cruz County for Louise's superb care.

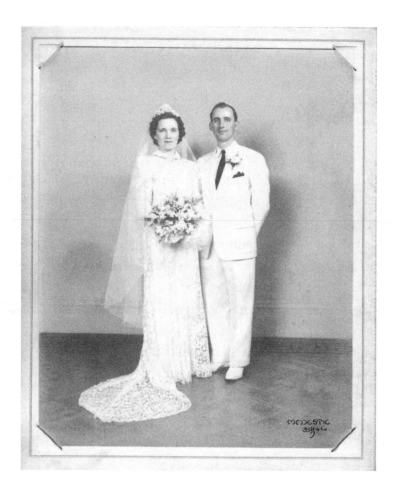

For Louise and Hank Wollenberg,
together again at last…

A Mother's Final Gift

Table of Contents

Foreword – George Daugherty

Emmy Award-winning producer, director, and conductor

EVERY HUMAN BEING ON OUR PLANET shares two momentous occasions: birth and death. In preparing for birth, there are great festivities, gifts are given, baby showers are planned and carried out, baptisms, brisos, and other religious rites are festively marked, nurseries are painted, cribs are built, booties are knitted, and the whole process is generally celebrated for nine months.

But death! Death is often another story. Most of us do not want to think about it – either about our own deaths, or the deaths of our loved ones. Death is the penultimate experience that will happen to all of us, and to everybody we know, but many of us become ostriches with our heads in the sand when faced with thinking about it. We often just ignore dealing with it.

This beautiful, touching book changed all of that for me. I had actually put off reading it because my own mother is ninety years old and not well. So at first, I was loath to read what I knew would be an emotionally-charged chronicle of another mother's death. But I did read it, and I feel exceedingly enriched and enlightened by having done so.

A Mother's Final Gift is the story of one courageous woman – Louise Viola Swanson Wollenberg – and of her tremendous love of life and family, and her faith and resolve. But it is also the story of her equally courageous family who, in the process of rising to the occasion and carrying out Louise's long-held final wishes, not only overcame so many stigmas about the process of death but, at the same time, rediscovered what it means to celebrate life itself.

This book not only touches the heart in a very powerful, poignant, and joyful way, but reading it was life-changing for me. In writing this book, Joyce and Barry Vissell, and their children, mentor us through an experience that many of us were afraid to even think about it. Louise looked at death as her greatest adventure. So should we all. The title of this book is indeed *A Mother's Final Gift* but, in truth, this story is an exceptional gift to every person who will read it.

Introduction – Barry Vissell

WE FEEL THAT MODERN SOCIETY'S ATTITUDES about dying need to change. Elizabeth Kubler-Ross, as well as other authors and researchers, have done much to bring dying out of the closet. But there is still much to be done. Too many dying family members are still put away in nursing homes, where they often are "out of sight and out of mind." They are also "out of heart," where the rest of the family misses out on an abundance of love and opportunities for personal and spiritual growth of the highest order.

We are a society still largely afraid of death. Modern medical science, while having done much to prolong and improve the quality of life, has also contributed to hiding death behind sterile walls, and removing death from homes. Many of us have given our authority over to medical institutions, assuming trained professionals know better than us how to help our loved ones die. But this is often not the case. We, as a medical doctor and nurse, as well as loving family members, want to bring dying back home where it belongs most of the time.

In indigenous cultures, as well as many other countries where medical science has not so clearly taken over, we still see people dying in the home, often with extended family living closely together. In these cultures, death is a natural phenomenon, not a medical procedure. The dying person is still part of the family, surrounded by the comings and goings of everyday living. Death is integrated into life, not separated from life.

No one understands this concept better than Hospice. This group of trained staff and volunteers has done more to bring dying back home than perhaps any other organization. Hospice was invaluable to our family in Louise's final months, allowing us to focus on our relationship with Louise rather than her medical management, allowing us to be with her, giving and receiving love, really learning from her dying.

Louise's feelings about dying remind me of so many stories about Native Americans and other indigenous peoples of the world. Death to many of these people is similarly not a scary thing, not something separate from life, to be hidden away in a dark closet. Dying is an integral part of living. It is, in fact, the ever-present awareness of death that allows for a fuller sense of life. It is the nearness of the old and the dying that helps to keep us aware of our own mortality, and hopefully the preciousness of life.

We predict, in the near future, there will be a flood of interest in keeping our loved ones home to die. As "baby boomers," we are already observing this great need in our society. Our parents have lived longer than their parents. And now they are dying, and we often have the means to take care of them in the most compassionate way.

Louise Wollenberg was not a saint with mystical powers or extraordinary spiritual gifts. Instead, she was a simple woman, mother, and grandmother who looked forward to her final adventure. She was not financially rich, but she was abundantly wealthy with the love of family and many friends. She took every opportunity to love those she knew — and to make new friends right up to the very days before her death.

Louise's last two weeks on earth were truly a mother's final gift. In those final days, she saw and spoke with beings that were invisible to the rest of us. She described events that eventually occurred at a future time. With our medical and psychiatric training, we could have easily passed this off as the hallucinations of a deteriorating mind. But we could not — not with Louise telling us things she couldn't possibly have known ahead of time. We were there. We saw the evidence.

This is not a book about how to care for a dying parent. It is a model to inspire other families to, whenever possible, keep their loved ones at home and to help them to die with dignity. It chronicles a mother and daughter's intimate dying experience, with all its mystery and miracles. It shows the ways that people — both those who are on their final journey, and the people who care for them—are transformed through the process of dying. The way Louise could communicate with unseen beings touched all of us in profound ways. When she saw or spoke with her "angels," the joy on her face was infectious, and the energy in the room felt different—more sacred.

When you are caring for someone who is dying, be prepared to be continuously surprised. Expect the unexpected. The outrageous often becomes the norm; it certainly did for us.

We hope this little book opens many eyes as well as hearts to this great need. We hope it inspires many more families to do what we did, to allow their loved ones to die with dignity in their own home. We hope this book will let readers know that they can both take care of their loved ones in the most compassionate way, and be transformed in the process. We also hope it will inspire people who dread death to instead look forward to an amazing adventure.

The Greatest Adventure of All

THREE WEEKS BEFORE SHE PASSED from this world, my ninety-year-old mother, Louise Viola Swanson Wollenberg, began what she called her "greatest adventure of all." It all started thirty-three years ago.

When I was twenty-seven years old, my mother came for a visit to our small rented home in Scotts Valley, California. One morning, she approached me and said, "Joyce, can we sit down together? I have something important to ask of you."

I remember every detail of this moment as if it were yesterday. I even remember the brown jumper I was wearing, and the way I kept twisting my five-year-old wedding ring upon my finger as she spoke. She spoke firmly but gently, "When it's my time to die, I want you to be excited for me. I'm not afraid to die. I feel that death will be my greatest adventure. When I lay dying, I want you to help me prepare for that great adventure. No matter how old I am, please know that I've had a good life and I'm grateful for all of it."

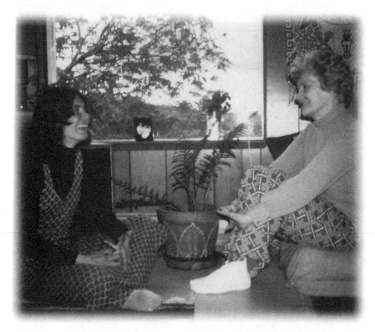

Barry sensed something important was happening, and
took this photo at the beginning of her talk.

I sat motionless, just staring at her, feeling that this
wasn't real. It just couldn't be possible that she had just
spoken those words. My mom was only fifty-six years
old, active and in perfect health.

I looked at her with a shocked expression and said,
"Mom, I could never be excited for you to die. That's
impossible!"

She smiled at me with compassion and said, "You're my daughter, and I know you'll find a way. I'm counting on you to be excited for me when I die."

Throughout the next thirty years, I contemplated her request. Sadness and an awful heaviness would flood my heart each time I thought about my mother dying.

When my mom was seventy-five years old and my dad was eighty-two, they moved into a little apartment above our garage at our new home near Santa Cruz, California, three thousand miles from their home in Buffalo, New York. Our three children were still living at home: Rami, sixteen; Mira, ten; and John-Nuri, three.

My dad died suddenly of a heart attack at age eighty-nine. We all felt devastated by the loss of a father and grandfather we loved and cherished and who had brought so much joy into our lives. My father's death made my attachment to my mother all the stronger. She and I spent at least an hour together every day and usually much more than that. She loved us all so much and loved everyone that came to see us. Every so often I thought of her request to me, made all those long years ago, that I be excited when it was her time to die. Each time the same thought came, "No, that's impossible. I couldn't possibly honor that request."

Nine years later, I found myself fully honoring my mother's request as she lay dying in her little apartment above our garage. Hospice had moved a hospital bed into the living room of this apartment where she had lived for fifteen years. The apartment was right next door to our family home, and held many happy memories of family gatherings for Saturday pancakes and birthday parties. My parents had shared this home for seven years before my father died. The last family celebration that he attended was their own sixtieth wedding anniversary.

One day as I walked into the apartment, my mom excitedly announced, "My angel came to me very early this morning when I woke up. I've always believed in angels, but for the first time in my life I actually saw one! She was radiant like the sun, and the whole room was filled with love and light."

My mother's face was still shining as she continued, "My angel told me that soon it'll be time for me to come back to my original home. She told me that I would be having wonderful and important experiences in the days before I died and she would be right here with me throughout the whole process. This is much more exciting to me than our trip to British Columbia or even my cruise to Sweden, my homeland. *This* will be my greatest adventure!"

Back home, I called our three children and asked them to come home for an important family meeting. That evening, sitting around our dining room table, I told them of Grandma's request that we be excited about her dying process. At first our children, like me so many years ago, were aghast at such a request, but then they began to understand that this was very important to their grandmother. We all committed ourselves to approach her bedside with enthusiasm about her next great adventure. We decided that if one of us was feeling sad or burned out, we would get help from the others.

With all the attention on Grandma's transition, our son wanted us to remember that in ten days he would be leaving home for college for the first time and wanted us to be excited for him as well. Two big transitions were happening at the same time. This was definitely a time of letting go. As we looked at each other that evening, we really had no idea of how deeply the next three weeks would impact our lives. They would be altered forever. We would never view death in the same way. As we gave my mother her final gift in honoring her dying process, she gave us her final gift of opening a window into eternity and allowing us to have a peek.

Over the next few weeks, our feelings soon turned into inspiration and awe as we each felt our lives being transformed by her dying process. None of us – Barry, Rami, Mira, John-Nuri or I – will ever be the same. We were allowed to be a witness to a sacred event, students in a miraculous schoolroom, as my mother communicated in her last three weeks all she was experiencing in her dying process.

This book is about one family's journey toward transformation, and the inspiration we all felt by witnessing the great and intimate passage called death. It is also about the conscious path of caring for an elderly family member, who for over a year was totally dependent upon us, incontinent, at times angry and unreasonable, at other times so sweet and loving that we, her family, were the recipients of her spiritual care. This book is about overcoming fears, doubts and self imposed limits. Indeed, it is about acquiring the courage to love more fully.

Our two daughters were 30 and 25 at the time and were fully involved in her day to day care. Our son was 17 and did what he could, with the small amount of time he had. Barry and I were both 60 years old, and changed more Depend Diapers in her last year than we ever thought possible.

With stunning clarity, she communicated to us in those last three weeks about where she was going, who she was seeing, how she was feeling, and the final instructions she was receiving. She saw and spoke of things that she couldn't have possibly made up. I sat, notebook in hand, and recorded it all, even though it would be three months after her death that I first had the idea to write this book.

Each of those final days, as she prepared for her greatest adventure, our whole family learned more about life and death, love and pain, confusion and certainty, and our excitement for her grew as well. My hope is that my mother's final gift, communicating and sharing the experience of her dying process, can bless your life as it has ours.

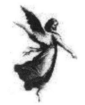

My mother was inspired when she talked about death. She was fascinated with the topic and read every book she could about death. She spoke about Elisabeth Kübler-Ross as if she were her best friend. For my mother, death was a glorious adventure. We all have an adventure or trip we dream about. Maybe we want to go to Africa and be with wild animals. Maybe we want to go to a tropical island and be totally alone. Barry wants the two of us to canoe the Yukon River in northern Canada for three weeks. For my mom, it was the adventure of death. She would talk about it the way someone might talk about a luxury cruise. Because she had no fear of death, she lived most of her life in a joyful, enthusiastic and grateful way.

My mother also had clear guidelines for us about her death. She did not want to have any extra procedures at the time of dying. She signed the form for DNR (Do Not Resuscitate.) She did not want to die in a hospital and did not want to be on pain medication to alter the natural process. It was extremely important to her that her wishes be honored. She often charged me with the responsibility of carrying out her wishes. Also, as she stated at age fifty-six, she wanted me to be excited for her to go on this exciting adventure.

When my mother talked about her own death, it drew the two of us very close. This may seem strange to some, but she was so inspired I couldn't help but be drawn into her enthusiasm. She was ever aware that death could come at any moment, as it had with her own mother, so she lived each day to the fullest. She reached out to people, made new friends and enjoyed whatever the day would bring.

A Mother's Promise

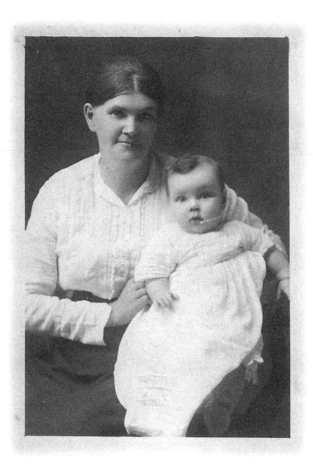

Baby Louise with her beloved mother, Amanda.

LOUISE VIOLA SWANSON WAS BORN in Westville, Pennsylvania on March 19, 1917—the seventh child of two Swedish immigrants. All seven children had been born at home with the help of a neighbor. On January 13, 1923, when Louise was six years old, her beloved mother, Amanda Swanson, had to be taken to the hospital because of weakness before giving birth to her eighth child. Louise, the youngest, was taken by train and ushered into the hospital room. Her mother opened her eyes when she heard the footsteps of her little daughter. Amanda reached out her hand to lovingly stroke Louise's head, and spoke gently, *"Everything will be all right. I am not afraid, dear Louisa. There's something I want you to always remember. I will NEVER leave you! Please, always remember this."*

Ten hours later Amanda died in childbirth while premature Betty lived. Louise was devastated. Later, when the open casket was set up in their small living room, she wanted to crawl right inside to be with her mother. Her coal miner father, Andrew, took her aside and said, "Your mother promised you she would never leave you. Now you must feel your mother, without being able to see her. Trust that she is always by your side. Live your whole life feeling your mother's love."

Those words set the course of my mother's life. She lived her entire life feeling the love of her mother as her best friend. Each day she would sit quietly and just feel that love. She knew her mother would be waiting for her when it was her time to pass from this world. Her mother passed from this world with grace and without fear. My mother wanted to do the same.

My parents lived to have sixty years of marriage. In the last five years of my dad's life, he and my mom

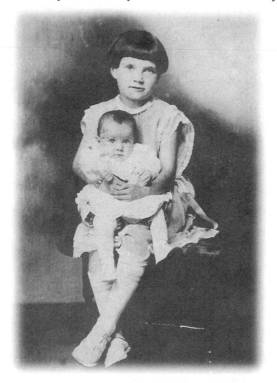

Louise with her baby sister, Betty, shortly after their mother's death.

VISSELL

began a ritual which they followed each evening before going to sleep. *They would say good-bye to each other.* They each knew that one of them could die in their sleep that night, for they both had heart disease. They would speak words of gratitude and affirmation that they would never be apart, even after death. When they both woke up the next morning, they were grateful to have the bonus of another day together. Their love and caring for one another was precious.

On August 21, 1999, Barry and I were coming back from a vacation with ten-year-old John-Nuri. While walking to the bathroom, my father had a massive heart attack and fell to the floor. Louise immediately called next door, where Rami and Mira happened to be at home. They both dropped everything and ran over to the apartment, where they quickly realized he was not breathing. Having recently taken a Red Cross course on CPR, they went right to work on him. Minutes later, the ambulance crew arrived and took over. Although they did everything they could, my father died enroute to the hospital, with my mom, Mira and Rami in the car behind the ambulance. The hospital set up a special room for them with my dad's body. They stayed there with his body for several hours. Rami told me that the hospital staff were very nice to them, especially a young nurse who kept bringing them water and tissues.

Several hours later, when Barry, John-Nuri and I returned home from our trip to British Columbia, we were met with the news. I burst into tears. My mother held me and kept saying, "If you were there when he died, you would know it was just so beautiful. We need to be happy for him."

A month later, we were giving a couple's workshop at a local retreat center. At dinner, Barry and I found ourselves sitting at a small table with two other couples we had never met before that weekend. I started telling them the story of my dad's death and how he was taken to Watsonville Hospital. One of the women at the table said, "Was your mother's name Louise, and was she with two granddaughters?"

"Yes," I immediately said.

"I was the nurse who took care of them."

I was surprised and happy to actually meet this woman by this amazing coincidence. She then related the following story: "I never saw anything like it before. Your mother did not cry or seem distressed. Her face glowed with acceptance. She wanted her granddaughters to know that death is a beautiful journey. She had them stroke your dad's skin to feel how soft it was, and all the while she was telling them that death is beautiful and needs to be welcomed and honored. At the hospital, we are used to tears, screams and stress, but not the peaceful scene that was happening around your dad. I kept walking in with water, tissues, and other things just because the energy was so special and I wanted to be close to them."

My mother's acceptance of my dad's death was so profound, I had friends visiting just to be around her because it felt so good. It seemed that a part of her was with her husband in that glorious heavenly place. It took me several months and many tears to be able to feel the same acceptance and realize my dad hadn't really gone anywhere. I could no longer see him, but I could still feel his love and devotion to the family. Sometimes I could almost hear the clomp, clomp, clomp of his shoes as he walked into our house and announced the mail.

Two years before he died, my dad built his dream workshop. He longed to work with his grandson there, but John-Nuri never seemed interested. About a year after Grandpa's death, John-Nuri asked for Barry's help with a school project that needed to be built in the workshop. For the very first time, John-Nuri was building something with Barry in Grandpa's special place. While they worked, all of a sudden an old alarm clock started ringing from a shelf above them. This was an old wind-up clock that my dad had in college, and only he could ever get it to work. After his death, it never worked again. As it was ringing, Barry and John-Nuri looked at one another in amazement and realized that Grandpa was there, happy to see his grandson in the workshop at last!

My mother and I enjoyed looking at pictures of Dad together, and there was always a happy tale to tell about each one. Through these pictures and memories, she was able to feel close to him each day of the eight years that she lived alone.

While you are reading about the beauty of my mother's death, it is also important to realize that she had prepared for her death from the time she was six years old and experienced her own mother's death. That experience was so transformative that she spent her whole life understanding and preparing for her own death and, in the process, prepared us for her absence. When her friends or seven siblings were approaching death, she tried to bring a positive attitude to the situation. Death was not some distant event to be dreaded. For my mother, her eventual death was something to be honored each and every day of her life.

The fact that she was almost totally helpless, sometimes in pain, and having to wear the "dreaded" adult diapers, did not take away from her experience. She constantly sought something deeper behind the pain and found love. From having both of her parents die at an early age, she knew life was not always fair. Just like a beautiful birth is often far from perfect, a beautiful death did not have to be pain-free or uncomplicated. She accepted the gift in just the way it was given.

Even though my mother prepared for her death from an early age, I believe that anyone at any stage in life can prepare for his or her death. In preparing oneself to have a positive attitude, the resources are there within us when this momentous time of our death is upon us. This attitude can be a tremendous gift and blessing to those who love and care for you. It is a gift of inspiration and modeling that lives on forever. I have learned many amazing and special things from my mother, but her attitude about death is what I most want to absorb into my heart and life.

Including Dying with Death
– Barry Vissell

UNTIL I ATTENDED MEDICAL SCHOOL, death was something I heard about, rather than witnessed. I remember playing in our back yard as a child when my mother came outside to tell me my grandma had just died. Although I loved my grandma, I didn't see her very often, and hadn't seen her sick with cancer. So it was just news. Bad news, but still news. It wasn't up close and personal.

In medical school, death and dying were clinical phenomena, to be studied in a detached intellectual way. The human cadaver my small group of first-year students and I dissected was only a real person in rare moments of reflection. The rest of the time it was organs, muscles and bones. Even the patients who died during my clinical rotations through the hospitals were often stripped of their humanity in our feverish attempts to prolong their lives.

Friends have died along the way, some closer to me than others, some very young. I was never present in the extremely intimate day-to-day dying process.

Then there was my own dad. One moment he was hugging my mom before she went out to do some errands. The next moment he sagged against her, falling over on top of her. Her first thought was that he was playing some sort of weird prank on her. Then she saw he was not breathing. By the time the first emergency team came to their house, ten minutes had elapsed and, although they restored his breathing and heartbeat, his brain had suffered irreversible damage.

I caught the first flight I could and arrived in San Diego that evening. My mom and I visited Dad in the hospital. He was connected to a breathing machine, and his heart was beating regularly with the use of drugs, but it felt to me like my dad was not there. His body lay in the hospital bed, blood and oxygen keeping it alive, but something vital and essential was gone. We went home for the night feeling the full weight of the decision we needed to make.

The next morning we arrived at the hospital and signed the forms to "unplug" his body, removing all machines and drugs. For the next hour, my mom and I watched his body gradually shut down as his breaths came with longer and longer intervals in between. My mom was stroking his head while she cried. I encouraged her to say good-bye, which she did. As he took his final breaths, I sang a song to him.

I distinctly remember I had no tears – until I called Joyce, minutes after his body was still. Then it felt like the floodgates opened, and the tears finally flowed.

Still, something was missing. It was death without dying. I missed the opportunity to say good-bye while my dad was still alive, to sit with him and integrate all the feelings of the dying process and, perhaps most of all, to listen to and feel his experience of dying.

Of course, over the years since his death I've had many conversations with my dad. I've said good-bye to him. I've expressed unfinished feelings and difficult realizations. And most importantly, I've expressed my love, which has given me the most peace. Still, it seems there will always be something missing around my dad's death.

I have received great gifts from Louise's dying process. Having her next door, seeing her every day, expressing my love to her, receiving her love, listening to her experiences, talking about death, all these things have changed my life for the better.

Louise gave me the gift of including dying with death. Death was no longer just news I received in the back yard of my childhood. It was a complex, dynamic, painful and joyful process, a life-changing experience. Death was part of living, not the end of living.

Dying is not neat; it's messy. I thought I would dread changing diapers on an old woman, or taking care of bedsores. Instead, it was something that needed to be done, and in fact could be done with tenderness and patience. Even the feelings are messy. I remember one day helping to move her body to relieve pressure on one of her bed sores. Louise screamed out in pain and anger, "You're torturing me." I found a capacity for patience that the closeness to death seemed to bestow upon me. I calmly said, "No, Louise, it just feels that way. Your bed sores will get worse if we don't move you."

Dying is not a clinical experience; it's extremely personal. I finally had the opportunity to turn off my "doctor mind," to stop trying to find solutions to her medical problems, to stop trying to figure out ways to prolong her life. Sometimes I wouldn't know how busy my mind was until I walked into Louise's apartment. It was like walking into a place where time simply didn't exist. The tranquility around her provided a stark contrast to my own lack of peace. It forced me to focus on my breathing, to calm myself down, so I could match her energy and connect heart to heart.

What an opportunity to silently look into Louise's eyes without any hesitation or embarrassment, to see her great serenity reflected in those luminous pools of light. Her eyes were truly the windows of her soul, and her soul was nearly always content with her current journey – except, of course, when she was in pain.

It was nearly impossible to gaze into those clear, shining eyes and not see the reflection of my own death, however far into the future. When I was really present with Louise, her dying was my dying as well. When I was at peace looking into her eyes, exchanging words of love, I was at peace with my own dying.

Louise knew with clear certainty that death was not the end of life. She knew death as the beginning, as well as part of, an even greater adventure and journey. Her calm certainty allowed those of us around her to touch our own knowing of life beyond the confines of the body. The times she spoke with her beloved Hank and other friends and family who had passed on, the things she shared with us about the world on the other side of the veil of death, were too inspiring not to be believed.

I suppose it would be possible to hang on to the belief that there is no life after death. But after sitting day after day with Louise, watching her body gradually shut down while watching something deeper and more essential actually getting stronger and more alive, witnessing a birth during the process of a death, how could anyone doubt the immensity and continuity of this journey? It feels to me the only way I could doubt life after death would have been to keep myself from looking into Louise's eyes, or listening to her wisdom and experience, or feeling the growing love in the room. I could only doubt the ongoing journey of her soul by refusing to see the birth happening in front of my own eyes.

Being with Louise's dying has allowed me to be with my living. Being with Louise's heart, her love and aliveness, has allowed me to be with my dying in a new way. When it is my time to die, I hope I am surrounded by the same love of family and friends, supporting me and helping me to launch into my next great adventure. I hope I can bring through wisdom from the next world to prepare the way for those after me. I hope I can inspire my family as much as Louise inspired all of us. I hope I can make my transition with the abundant expectancy I witnessed in Louise.

Like an Old Clock

PEOPLE OFTEN ASK US, "What disease did Louise have?" We have to answer she didn't die from any particular disease. Her heart disease was not the cause of her death. She died because it was the right time for her. Her whole body was shutting down, like an old clock slowly winding down, rather than any particular organ system failure. She gradually lost the ability to walk by herself, feed herself, use the bathroom, and be independent in any way. Her appetite, and finally her thirst mechanism, simply faded away.

Our family is vegetarian and very health conscious. We try to eat as much raw food as possible. I never forced my diet on my mom. She cooked meat, used dairy products, and ate the way she always ate, even in her elderly years. I did give her a lot of healthful supplements, like blue-green algae in tablet form. She took all these things, perhaps to humor me or maybe she understood that they really were helping. I always made my mom fresh carrot, celery and beet juice, which she enjoyed very much. There was never a fight about this.

One year before she died, she suddenly refused to drink any of the vegetable juices I made for her each day. We got into heated discussions, with me telling her she must, and she telling me she wouldn't. Well, she won. One by one, she stopped eating anything healthy, except the supplements.

"I want to eat what I want to eat," she stubbornly asserted. At this point, my mom was not able to go to the grocery store and shop for herself. She was dependent upon us. It felt terrible to all five of us to give her food we knew was not healthy for her. We tried the old disciplinary technique of eat your vegetables first and then you can have a cookie. It didn't work. She just refused to eat and was losing weight daily.

Finally, we had to surrender. I bought the food she wanted. Cookies, ice cream, candy and watermelon (the only healthy item she liked) became her diet. She was happy, though. In time, even these foods were not interesting to her. She went from weighing 130 to 100 pounds in six months.

Three weeks before my mom died, she was moved into a hospital bed. The Hospice nurse had a meeting with me about my mother's condition. With so much kindness, she looked at me and said, "Your mother's skin is breaking down. This is the largest organ in the body. Even with the best care, she is getting bed sores. It probably will get worse."

Our family had a conference and decided that if Grandma asks for something to eat or drink, try to distract her once. If she could be distracted, then she wasn't really hungry. If she asks again, then give her whatever she wants. In the two weeks before she died, she only asked for sips of water.

She became incredibly clear. Her eyes shown brilliantly and her mind was clear. She was as much a part of the heaven world into which she was entering as she was a part of our world. She was getting ready to go back to her true home. Her long-term memory became very clear, and she was able to convey to us all she was experiencing. Rather than these two weeks being a sad and gloomy time, it was inspiring and exciting for all of us. Each day we would wake up wondering what amazing lesson she was going to give us that day. Through her communications to us, she shared every step of her dying process. We, in turn, were drawn into the spiritual energy she was living so fully.

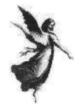

Barry's note: Four days before Louise died, I was sitting with her when suddenly she said, "Barry, I would love some ice cream right now."

I was surprised because she hadn't eaten a thing in about a week and a half. Nevertheless, I ventured over to her freezer and found a small container of chocolate ice cream, her favorite. Bringing it to her bedside, I touched a teaspoon to the ice cream so that a small part of the spoon had barely enough to give a hint of taste. As the spoon approached her open mouth, Louise looked delighted. I touched the spot of ice cream to her waiting tongue and she closed her eyes, savoring the experience. After a while she spoke, "That was delicious!"

"Do you want some more, Grandma?"

"No, thanks. That was enough."

First Visit with Dad – August 13

MONDAY, AUGUST 13, 2007, thirteen days before her death, my mom finally saw her beloved husband again. The day was beautiful, and she had had a cluster of visitors, some of her very favorite people. She sat like a queen on a throne, while we all sat around her hospital bed. She joked with us and was the life of the party. Our friend Charley Thweatt sang to her, and she loved it. Charley is a very talented singer and songwriter whose music has added much depth to our work with groups. My mother has always had a crush on him, often referring to him as her "boyfriend," even though he is thirty-five years younger than she is. He goes along with the joke and calls her "his darling."

After everyone left, she fell into a peaceful sleep. I went to check on her several hours later and just sat quietly with her. It had become my habit to have a notebook and pen with me. I didn't want to forget anything she said.

Suddenly, she opened her eyes and focused right above her. Tears started flowing from her eyes, and she said, "Hank, I can see you again. You look so beautiful, just like the day we got married so long ago. I've so missed being able to see you. How is it that you look so much younger, while I have so many more wrinkles? You are my beloved. I've never stopped loving you and thinking about you."

Then there was a period of silence during which she was slowly nodding her head in agreement. Finally, she spoke again to him. "Hank, I'm so happy I'm coming home to you very shortly. I'll do as you told me and say good-bye to everyone. Please tell me what our new home is like."

There was another long silence while my mother smiled and listened attentively. Her face full of rapture, she said, "Oh, I always felt it would be that wonderful."

There was a brief period of silence which was followed by my mom saying, "Yes, there is something that still bothers me, and I can't seem to find the gift behind it. I just don't understand why Joyce took away my driver's license. I was such a good driver, and I never had an accident or received a ticket. I have accepted so many things that have happened to me, but this just seemed so unfair. It hurt my feelings, and I can't seem to let it go."

I thought to myself, "Oh no, here we go again…"

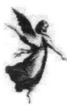

When my mom was eighty-six, her driver's license expired and she needed to take the written test once again. She took the test twice and failed miserably. She was discouraged because she really wanted to continue driving. I knew she was a good driver and could see how much joy and independence it brought her. So, for months after the failed tests, I coached her every evening on the rules of driving. I made cards for her and asked her to go over them each day: How long does a child need a car seat? What alcohol blood level is considered a DUI? These and other answers my mother didn't need to know except to pass her test. We went over and over these things each night, and the following day they would be forgotten, because she simply had no use for the information.

Finally, I felt she was prepared and took her myself for the test. She failed again. I told the woman she is a good driver, who only goes a few miles on side roads to the beach, grocery store and her church. She gave us one more month to study, and said she could have an in-person test.

She and I studied and everyone she knew was praying for her. Finally she got the blood alcohol content correct and remembered that a child needs to be six years old or weigh sixty pounds before they can be out of a car seat. She dressed in her prettiest clothes, had her hair done, and then was ready to take the final test. If she failed, she could never drive again. She sat across from the woman asking the questions, and I watched her flash her winning smile and treat yet another person like she was an old friend.

She passed! For three more years she was a safe driver in her little red car, managing to completely avoid the freeway.

Barry and I were leading a workshop in New Jersey when the call came from our son that Grandma's car had been stolen. Why would anyone steal her little old Toyota Tercel? It was hardly worth anything. Apparently, my mother had gone to her old hairdresser, rather than the new one with whom she had an appointment. They knew her well and did her hair even though she didn't have an appointment. When my mother couldn't find her car in the large parking lot, the kind hairdresser drove her home. Assuming that Grandma just couldn't find her car in the parking lot, our three children and Rami's boyfriend, River, went looking for it. However, they went to the parking lot of the new hairdresser, where Grandma had actually *had* the appointment. She forgot to tell them she went to the old hairdresser. When they could not find the car, they called the police.

A policewoman came to my mom's apartment and began filling out a report. She sent out an alert for the "stolen car." An hour later, the police found the car, right in the parking lot of the hairdresser who had actually done her hair. It had been untouched, just sitting awaiting my mother's return.

The policewoman who came to make the report asked to speak with our children and River. She went outside with the four of them and, in a quiet voice, told them she was in charge of the area where my mother usually drives. She had noticed her over the years and always felt that she was a safe driver. But in the last few months, she witnessed my mom driving too slowly and having difficulty with intersections. She felt it was time for my mom to stop driving. She said either we take her license away or she would. Then she looked at our children as she said, "It's very embarrassing for an elderly person to have the police take away their license. Why doesn't the family do it?"

Two days later I was back home. I had my mom take me for a ride and saw for myself that it was time to take away her license. Afterwards, I pointed out all the potentially dangerous mistakes she had made. I gently reassured her that it was time to let other people drive her around. I assured her I would set up rides for her whenever she wanted to go somewhere. Then I took away her car keys. My mom could never accept this. She maintained she was a good driver and insisted I had no reason to take her license away. She told me that everyone loses their car sometimes and why should she have to be punished. She evidently didn't get the message that she was not a safe driver.

In all fairness, I understand how difficult this can be. For so many seniors, driving their own car is a powerful symbol of their independence. It is for this reason that many seniors drive longer than they should.

My mother was embarrassed to tell the truth to her close friends who were still driving, so she began making up stories which always made me sound like the bad guy. "I was driving down our little private road and someone else hit me. Joyce came running down the hill and took away my license, when it wasn't my fault at all."

The stories changed daily, but one fact remained in her mind: she was a good driver, and I shouldn't have taken away her license. I asked my brother Bruce to explain it to her. Bruce has always held a lot of authority in my mom's life, plus she loves him dearly.

Surely he could explain it. She accepted his answer for a few days and then was back to her theory of it being entirely my fault.

I then spoke with her minister, Bob Bowles, whom she absolutely adores. Bob sat down with her and gently explained it wasn't my fault. That lasted maybe an hour, then it was back to it being my fault and she should be allowed to drive.

At first, I was upset at hearing these stories over and over again. Each visitor to her home heard one version or another. Eventually, I just began to accept that perhaps she would carry this to her death. On the whole, our relationship was very harmonious, and this was the only point of strife. I tried to see it as humorous, but never quite could, as the stories always made me sound like a mean daughter. I wished my mother would understand that I had only taken the keys away for her safety.

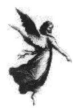

After my mom asked my dad, "Why did Joyce take away my driver's license?" there was a long silence. I waited anxiously. Could my dad answer this question for her? No one else had been able to get her to understand.

Finally she spoke, and I held my breath, "Oh ... I understand now. I see what happened. Joyce had no other choice. I've been blaming her all this time. You're right, I need to apologize to her."

That was the end of her first visit with my dad. She closed her eyes for awhile. When she next opened them, she excitedly said, "Joyce, I finally got to see Dad again. He looks fantastic! I'm so thrilled to be going to be with him. I'm so sorry for blaming you for taking away my driver's license. I just never understood until Dad explained it to me."

The subject of her driver's license never came up again. Dad had been able to get through to her when the rest of us could not—as he always had been able to do—and, as usual, he spoke to her matter-of-factly. It was so much his style that I did not doubt that she had actually been talking with him.

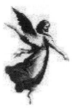

My mother and father were deeply in love with each other. Shortly before my dad passed away, they celebrated their sixtieth anniversary. The love and devotion between them was beautiful to behold. My parents definitely had their share of challenges and difficulties in their relationship, but they were happiest in their last twenty years.

Five years before my dad passed away, he lost all of his hearing. There could be a loud crash behind him, and he wouldn't hear it. To communicate with him, we wrote notes, and he answered with a booming voice that sometimes startled us. He couldn't hear anyone speak, yet for some odd reason he could often understand my mom. It seemed that he was hearing her with his heart rather than his ears.

I worried my mom would feel a deep loneliness and despair after his passing. Her life had revolved around my dad. Since he couldn't hear, she drove him places, took him out to lunch almost every day, fixed meals for him, and in general fussed over him in every detail. Instead, over the following months and years until she joined him, she loved to sit alone in my dad's favorite place on the couch. When I would go to check on her, she would be sitting quietly with a smile upon her face. When I'd ask her what she was doing, she would reply, "I'm just having a nice time with Dad."

Curious, I'd ask, "Do you see him?"

"No, but I can sure feel him. He's just pouring his love upon me, waiting for me to join him." She never wavered from that peaceful acceptance, knowing her beloved husband, Hank, was waiting for her.

In the months before her death, she would ask me to hold up my dad's picture while she was lying in bed, ready for sleep at night. As I held it up, she would say, "Hold on Hank, I'm coming soon. I need to go to John-Nuri's graduation, and then I'll be joining you." After John-Nuri's graduation, she would say, "Hank, I'm just about there. Ann is coming with Emily, and I must wait and see them. (Ann was my brother's first child who lived in Philadelphia and Emily her daughter.) After that visit, she found out my brother was coming for the three weeks our family had to be away working, so she would say, "Hank, just one more visit. I'd like to stay and be with Bruce one last time, and Allen (my brother's oldest son) is coming too. Just keep holding on. I'm packing my bags. I can't wait to see you again. I just really want to have these family visits."

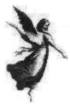

Since my mother's mother had died at such an early age, she was always imagining that someone else could be her mother. When she was nineteen years old, she found the perfect woman in her church. This woman and her husband would come into church fashionably dressed, and always sat in the same pew. My mother would then slip in behind her and imagine she was sitting right behind her mother. This went on for months.

Meanwhile, a friend had arranged a blind date for my mother and her best friend, Dorothy. The two young men, who had been away at college, were going to come in separate cars to pick up my mom and Dorothy. Dorothy was a bit bossy, so she said to my mother before the men showed up, "I'm older than you, so I get the guy with the nicer car." My mother, who came from a very poor family, did not mind at all. The guy in the nicer car, Harlow, became Dorothy's husband. The guy in the poorer car, Henry, became my dad.

My dad instantly fell in love with my mom and wanted his parents to meet her. Well, I guess you can imagine the end of this story. My dad's mother was the same lady that my mother had been sitting behind in church all those months! At last, my mother had a mother again – and a wonderful man who became her husband two years later.

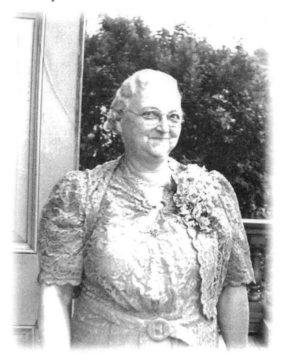

Hank's mother, so happy to see her son marrying Louise.

She Believed in my Life – August 14

OUR LONG-TIME FRIEND AND MUSICIAN, John Astin, came to sing to Mom today. John is a very gifted musician, and his songs go right to the heart. My mother has always loved him over the years. He sang several beautiful songs for her and ended with a special song in honor of her journey:

"Blessings on your journey
blessings on your way
on your way back home
just carry the light within you
just carry the light within you."

Throughout this song, she closed her eyes and had the most beautiful smile on her face. When John was done singing she opened her eyes, thanked him and said, "I am enjoying my journey back home. This will be the best journey I've ever taken." She then closed her eyes and slept peacefully.

I let my mother sleep the rest of the day. I checked on her every hour. She was always in the same deep sleep. She loved to have the visitors, since she loved people so much. However, I found she needed more and more time alone. She seemed to be preparing herself for her journey.

That evening, our family had dinner together. This was a dinner with mixed emotions. Since my dad died eight years ago, the six of us had spent a lot of time together. Now, John-Nuri would be leaving for college in just two days and we were realizing this would be the last time the five of us could be together with Grandma. She was still sleeping from the morning, but I decided it was more important to wake her up and have a short time with the six of us still together.

It was the family's idea to go over and sing to her. She loves when we do this. Like little angels, we crept around her bedside and very softly began singing to her.

She opened her eyes, looked confused to see us, and said, "I was just having the most delightful visit with Hank." Then she closed her eyes again. When she next opened them, a look of disappointment spread across her face as she said, "He's gone. We were having so much fun together."

Then she seemed to understand she was still in her body, and her family had come to sing to her. "Oh, please sing my Louise song." We sang to her for about half an hour and she seemed to love it. Then she sweetly said, "I've been keeping Dad waiting long enough. I'd like to go back to him."

The rest of the family tiptoed out of the room while I remained. She lay still for a while, then a huge smile spread across her face as she enthusiastically spoke: "I'm so glad you came back, Hank!" There was mostly silence on her part, but every once in a while she would say a short phrase like, "Oh, really! Oh, that sounds lovely! I can't wait to join you. Oh my, it must be so wonderful and beautiful. I am so happy to be joining you soon."

After a while, there was only silence. She had the most contented look upon her sleeping face. I stayed in the room just looking at her and reflecting on how grateful I felt to have been able to care for her this past year and now to be able to be with her in her dying process.

Some people had been critical of me for keeping my mother home when she developed so many disabilities, like losing all bladder and bowel control, and only walking with assistance. They felt I should put her in a nursing home and move on with my life. They argued that I was spending too much time caring for her and added, "Yes, we know you love your mother. But once a person can't use the bathroom by themselves, it is time to put them in a nursing home where they have round-the-clock care. You can't put your life on hold just because your mother is failing." These comments and lack of support hurt my feelings, but they never deterred my commitment to keep her home where I knew she felt safe and secure. My mother had always been there for me and I wanted to do the same for her.

Sitting next to her while she lay so peacefully, I thought of a time over forty years ago when I was twenty years old and almost died in a New York City hospital. I was a first year nursing student at Columbia University and was visiting Barry at his parent's home an hour north of the city. I developed a toothache and needed to have an emergency dental appointment with Barry's family dentist. It turned out to be a large tooth abscess, which he had to open up to drain. He neglected to give me antibiotics. Barry then dropped me off in New York City and returned to school in Boston.

The next day, I developed septicemia, a massive infection in my bloodstream. My temperature soared to over 106 degrees. I was quickly admitted into the university hospital, where antibiotics failed to bring down the fever. In a desperate measure, I was wrapped in ice and put in a cooling tent.

I remember looking up at all the doctors and nurses in the isolation intensive care unit. They all looked so worried as they hurried around me doing various procedures. I remember thinking to myself, "My body feels so terrible. It would be so much easier to just let go and leave this world." I then lapsed into a coma.

A doctor called my parents and told them, "If you wish to see your daughter alive, you need to come right away. We are not sure she will live."

It was almost December, and Buffalo was experiencing blizzard conditions. There was only one plane scheduled to fly to New York, and there was only one seat on that plane. My parents decided my mother should have that seat.

My mother finished her duties as church secretary and hurried home to get ready for the flight. Another call from the nursing school confirmed there was little chance I would be alive by the time my mother arrived.

By the time my mother sat on the plane and buckled her seat belt, she was hit by the full reality of what was happening. I might be dead by the time she got to me. She told me later she knew she could respond one of two ways. Part of her felt like melting into a puddle of tears, but a stronger part of her knew she must place my life in the hands of God. She told me she bowed her head in prayer and fully entrusted God with my life. She promised to accept God's will for my life. As she did so, she later told me, "I felt as if Jesus himself came and sat down next to me. He told me to not worry. He was right here. For my entire flight to New York, I felt enveloped in the most love and peace I have ever felt."

When my mother arrived at LaGuardia Airport, it was late at night and snowing heavily. There was a line of cabs waiting to take customers into the city. Columbia Presbyterian Hospital was a short ride, and the cab drivers all wanted a long ride to make more money, since the airport was closing. The whole long line of cab drivers refused to take my mother. At the very end of the line she came to an older African-American cab driver. My mother had always been a strong civil rights activist, and this was 1966, a time of unrest among African-Americans. This man offered to take her to the hospital and, when he found out I was possibly dying, sang gospel songs and prayed with her. At the end of the ride, he refused to take any money. I sometimes wonder if that man was perhaps an angel in disguise.

The director of the nursing school met my mother's cab and escorted her directly to my hospital room. It felt like I was not in my body, for I strangely remember looking down and seeing every detail of my mother approaching my room, even though the room door was closed. Outside the room there was a circle of about eight doctors. The hospital had called not only the experts from Columbia University Hospital but also experts from Cornell Hospital. An older man, probably the attending physician, approached my mother and respectfully said, "We're sorry, Mrs. Wollenberg. We have done all we can and have brought in the top experts in the city. Your daughter is dying and there is nothing we have been able to do about it. Do you want me to walk in with you? Your daughter does not look the same way as when you last saw her."

I then heard my mother say, "No, I want to go in by myself." She told me later she was still feeling the same loving presence that surrounded her on the plane. She said, "Though they told me you were dying, this presence of love told me it was not so. I felt full confidence you would live."

When my mother touched the handle of the door and began to open it, I suddenly came back into my body. As she entered the room, a ray of bright light came into my heart and I was instantly alert, after having been in a coma for over twelve hours. She walked over to my bed and took my hand and simply said, "Hi, Sis. You're going to be all right now."

I weakly replied, "Oh, Mother, I need you so much. Thank you for coming."

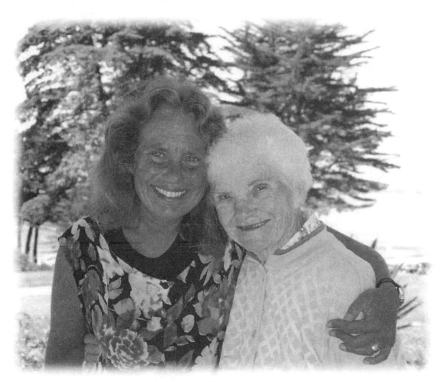

I began to get better from that moment on. It took several weeks, but my mother's appearance was the turning point from near death to life. I believe my mother brought me back to life by her total surrender to God's will and a belief in my life.

My mother stayed at my side and helped me to begin eating, walking and all the aspects of starting to get strong again. After one week, I ordered my mother to go back home. I was not even very nice about it. I felt horrible after she left and called to tell her I was sorry. I didn't know why I had done that. I believe I had been so uncomfortable about needing my mother so much, I was trying to prove to myself I didn't need her as much as I did. I missed her so much after she left. As I grew just a bit older, I came to peace with how much I needed my mother's love.

Now sitting in her room, watching her dying process, I felt how I would always need my mother's love. I closed my eyes and realized that even when I could no longer see her or hear her voice, I would feel her enduring love within my heart.

Keeping My Mother Home – August 15

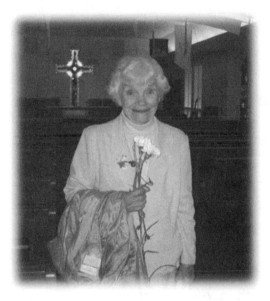

MY MOTHER BELONGS to the St. Andrew Presbyterian Church in our little community of Aptos. It is a small congregation of mostly white-haired people who deeply care about one another. Until two years ago, my mother was in charge of sending out weekly letters to the "shut-ins," those unable to come to church in person. She would hand me her manually-typed letter and ask me to "mimeograph" it. (Technology just wasn't her thing.) Even when she became a shut-in herself, she was still thinking about the shut-ins that seemed more shut-in than she was. She would send them little cards or pray for them daily. She never quite accepted that now she was one of them.

My mother loved hymns, especially "How Great Thou Art," and she loved the Hallelujah Chorus from Handel's *Messiah*. Music would put her in such a special place that tears would come into her eyes. I believe she loved music so much because her clearest childhood memory was of her mother singing these sacred songs.

I called her church and asked for people to come and sing to her. On this warm, sunny day, a lovely man named John came to sing hymns to her. He was one of the soloists in the church choir and had a beautiful, strong voice. Mother was in bliss while he was singing. He stayed for almost an hour, singing any hymn she wanted. Of course, he had to sing "How Great Thou Art" several times.

After he left, she closed her eyes, and a look of complete contentment was upon her face. She did not appear to be sleeping (as she snores softly when asleep), but seemed to be in another world, listening intently to something I couldn't hear. I sat with her for quite a while. Every once in a while, she would say things like, "This music is even better than John." Or,

"Not even Ruth (her daughter-in-law) can sing like this." "Oh, this is the best music I have ever heard."

When she opened her eyes and registered my presence in the room, she said, "The music where I'm going is so special. I've never heard anything more beautiful. John and Ruth sing so beautifully, and you know my favorite singing voice of all is John-Nuri, but none of them can compare to the music from where I'm going." Then she smiled at me sweetly and said, "I'm so excited to be going to my new home!"

Since my husband and I are medical professionals, we could have attributed my mother's experiences to a drug reaction. But she had been adamant that she wanted to experience this journey drug-free, and we had honored that request. We could have also blamed a deteriorating mind, but she clearly was present and very aware. In some ways, she was more present and aware during the times when she was having these contacts with a non-physical realm.

With bright shining eyes, my mother looked at me and said, "Joyce, I'm so happy you are allowing me to stay in my own home. I feel so peaceful here with all my family pictures and happy memories. In the quiet of this room I can focus upon where I'm going." She once again closed her eyes and the same look of contentment spread across her face.

Sitting next to her, I reflected on how it came to be that we were able to keep my mother home. It was hard to watch her slow decline, which all happened in the last year of her life. She had always been so active, walking a mile on the beach each day, gardening, cooking and baking for her grandchildren, and caring for "shut-ins." I first became aware of my mother's decline when I noticed a pile of wet clothes hidden in her closet, smelling of urine. She stopped making her bed and, when I made it each morning, I would typically discover a wet spot. At first I just took care of everything in secret, not wanting to embarrass her. Eventually she started waking up totally wet, and it was time to address the issue.

About fourteen months before my mother died, she needed adult diapers. I knew such things existed, but I had never before seen one nor knew how to use them. I now consider myself to be an expert. My mother did not like to wear her diapers. She'd pull them off at night and I'd come in and find the bed all wet again. Her innocent reply was, "Oh, they must have fallen off." Well, I knew they didn't fall off. It was time for a confrontation. We had a long talk about this. After telling her how hard it was for me to change her bed each day, she finally consented and wore the diapers until the day she died.

She had always gone to my brother's house for the summer and wanted to go again. My brother Bruce and his wife Ruth are very caring and loving people. My mother loves them and their four children and grandchildren very much. My brother and his wife felt that when Mom started having bowel movements in her diapers, it was time to put her in a nursing home. Most people believe the same. No one wants to change smelly, messy diapers on an adult. I changed thousands of diapers on our three children, but changing an adult was a totally different experience.

This was the time to really evaluate if we could keep her at home with us. I looked at a few nursing homes and felt really depressed when I came home. The patients were crowded into colorless, uninteresting rooms. In the noisy atmosphere, I just didn't see genuine loving and caring from the staff. Did I really want to come to a nursing home each day to be with my mother, or did I want to keep her at home and visit her in the beauty of her own surroundings?

Just because her diapers are smelly and messy, does that mean we need to kick her out? Once again our family had a conference.

Rami, Mira, Barry and I then had a long talk and, at the end, agreed to give it a try to keep Grandma home, which meant tackling those dirty diapers. So, for ten months, until she died, we changed her diapers. Since we had different shifts, one of us might get lucky and not have to do the messy part for several days. But then there was usually a challenging situation that awaited us the next time we did. None of us ever got to the point where we could say we enjoyed that part of her care, but our enjoyment of having her home with us more than made up for this inconvenience.

John-Nuri agreed to take Grandma back and forth to her church every Sunday (as long as he didn't need to stay) and take her on as many walks to the beach as he could.

Almost all of our friends came forth with great help. Some brought her homemade cookies each week (her favorite food). Others came and sang. Some came and just sat and talked with her. All of the people that came to help were so grateful for the opportunity to be with her.

I have made several really good decisions in my life. Of course, my spiritual decisions are the most important. After that, the next best decision was marrying Barry and having our three children. Next was our choice of service and work. And the next in importance was keeping my mother home. Though initially we received very little support for our decision, it proved to be the best decision ever. She felt so secure and so loved in her own home, and through that security and love she was able to give us her great gift: a model of dying consciously and without fear.

Barry, Rami, Mira, John-Nuri and I did all we could to make her comfortable and happy, and she thrived under our love. Yes, we each sacrificed in that year we cared for her. Yes, Barry and I were not able to do as many of our workshops as we normally do, and our finances suffered somewhat because of it. Yes, we all missed out on some fun activities and trips. But that sacrifice has turned into a warm glow within our hearts whenever we think of that time. Not one of us has regrets, wishing we would have given her more attention or love. We each gave fully of ourselves, and that knowledge brings a beautiful peace.

Four months before my mother died, I was beginning to feel the strain and responsibility of caring for her in addition to working perhaps thirty hours a week. Rami, Mira and Barry were helping regularly with her care, and John-Nuri helped on Sundays. I felt very grateful for all the help, but I personally carried the ultimate medical and emotional responsibility. Our children could go off and live their lives and forget about Grandma when it was not their turn to care for her. This was good and what I wanted. However, I never could forget. Barry helped me a lot, but in order for me to concentrate more on my mother, he had to take on most of the office work. The responsibility began to feel like a weight I was carrying. Each day this weight seemed heavier and heavier. One week I cried every day. It hurt to see my once vital and energetic mother becoming weaker and frailer. She was losing weight every day and her skin was breaking down and healing poorly.

One morning, I woke up and just started crying. I just didn't feel like I could continue taking care of my mother. Later, I was walking our dogs on our country road when our neighbor, Kathy Tucker, a former Hospice nurse, slowly drove by. She stopped to ask how my mother was doing. After I told her, she replied, "You need to call Hospice. They'll be a wonderful support for you."

"Hospice?" I felt shocked by her suggestion. "But my mother is not dying next week. She could even live a few more years."

"Hospice will come. The only requirement is that your mother is declining," Kathy went on to explain. "Has she been losing weight?"

"Yes, steadily," I answered.

"Well, that's all Hospice needs."

After she drove away, I rejected the idea immediately, as it seemed almost cruel to my mother. I felt if

I called Hospice, I would be telling her she was going to die soon, which at the time didn't seem imminent.

A week went by, and the weight of the responsibility of my mother's care seemed heavier than ever. Each morning when I awoke, I challenged myself to not cry that day, to try and make it through just one day without tears. While walking our dogs, Kathy Tucker again pulled up to talk. After finding out about my mother, she again asserted, "You really should call Hospice. They will be an amazing support for you. And your mom's insurance will cover the entire cost." The idea was not so easily rejected this time. She had used the magic word "support," the one thing I was absolutely craving.

That night I sat alone and stared at the Hospice phone number. It took me an hour to get up the courage to call. Calling Hospice would mean my mother was dying, and I would have to fully admit that to myself and then tell her. Finally, at seven that evening, I dialed the phone. I felt that probably they would be closed, and I could just leave a message. Then, when they called back, I could ignore it if I wanted.

The most wonderful, caring voice picked up my call and said, "Hospice of Santa Cruz County." My eyes filled with tears at the compassion in this woman's voice. With her first spoken words, I felt I had entered into the most caring, supportive environment there could possibly be for me right then. I felt God speaking to me in my heart saying, "This is the answer to your prayer. You can trust these people."

I briefly told the woman I just wanted information, and she asked me to hold on for a minute. In just a few seconds, the evening admitting nurse was on the phone. I had only wanted to leave a message, and here I was talking to the admitting nurse. The reality of what I was doing set in, and the tears started flowing. The nurse spoke gently and with compassion, "We know how very hard this first call is. Tell me about your mother. I have all the time you need."

For over an hour, I poured my heart out to this nurse. I told her about my mother, but I also told her about my struggles and how I felt this heavy weight from carrying all the responsibility for her care. I cried and she listened without interruption. Even on the phone, I felt as if I had crawled into the lap of a compassionate mother, and she was soothing me with her listening as well as her words. She explained Hospice is not just for people who are dying immediately. It is for people who are declining, like my mother. Hospice will take them on for six months. If they are getting better in six months, then Hospice steps away. I knew deep down my mother would not be getting better.

The nurse also explained that my mother's insurance would cover every aspect of her Hospice care. However, in signing on for Hospice, I would have to also decline her hospital insurance privileges. Knowing how much my mother hated hospitals, and had begged me to never take her to a hospital again, this was not a difficult decision. The nurse told me my first step was to go to my mother's physician and ask him to release her into the care of Hospice. There were also many forms he would have to sign. This nurse told me they were there to help and support me in my process with my mother. Those words soothed me to the very core of my being. I desperately needed help and support.

The next day a different Hospice nurse called and asked if she could come over that day. I happened to have time in the afternoon and she worked around my schedule. I also asked if I could talk to her in private before we went up to see my mother. When she arrived, I ushered her into our house and told her I didn't know when my mother would die, and wanted her to present Hospice in a way that didn't make it seem as if she were dying next week. The nurse smiled and said she knew just how to do that.

We then went up to see my mother together. The nurse was very skilled and by the end of the visit my mother said, "I'm so happy you're here to help my daughter with my care. She's seemed worried lately."

Before Hospice, I felt like I was carrying a heavy responsibility all by myself. With Hospice, it felt like many legs came to support the same table. My mother had Carol, her very own wonderful nurse who would be in charge of all of her medical concerns. Carol would visit every week, and more if necessary. We also had Lara, a social worker who was very supportive to both my mother and me. We elected to have Emily, a chaplain who would come every week and support her spiritually. Hospice chaplains are trained to be with people of all faiths and support them as they are able, always aiming for what brings meaning and comfort for them.

She was also sent Susie, a home health aide who would come three times a week and give her a shower, wash her hair or whatever else my mom needed. As my mother declined, Susie came five mornings a week.

Hospice further sent a volunteer, a man in his forties named Mark. For several months, Mark was such good medicine for my mother. He came two days a week and took her for a walk on the beach in her wheelchair. Then he took her out for ice cream and usually bought flowers at the florist for her. My mother considered this a "date," and always wanted to get all dressed up for "Mark Days." The fact that Mark was fairly young, (half my mother's age), and in her own words, "very handsome," made her feel quite special. Mark Days were always looked forward to. He had gone through the Hospice volunteer training program and knew just how to treat my mother. She loved him and all the attention he gave her. When she could no longer leave her apartment, he sat by her bed and told her all about golf tournaments. She had loved golf up until the age of seventy-six.

Hospice also supplied all the medicines, lotions, shampoos, creams and diaper pads that my mother needed. If Carol felt Louise needed a certain medicine, supplement or piece of equipment, she would call and it was sent usually within the day, often within the hour. The communication system between all those involved in my mother's care was so exact; I never had to worry about information lapses. Everyone on her team knew what was going on.

I started walking with a lighter step. Before, I was trying to do it all, and now my only concentration was on loving and enjoying my mother. If something went wrong, I simply called Hospice and they either answered my question by phone or sent someone right away. I have often reflected that Hospice people are some of God's most loving angels here on earth. They are so filled with compassion and understanding. It seems their mission is to bring dignity and comfort to the dying process, for both the person dying and the family members caring for that person. Calling Hospice early on in my mother's process was indeed a great blessing and one of the very best things I did both for my mother and for myself. Help and support were now in abundance, 24/7.

How a Son-in-law Became a Son
– Barry Vissell

WHEN JOYCE FIRST STARTED DATING, her dad took her aside and said, "I don't care who you date as long as he's not Jewish and doesn't come from New York City."

Undoubtedly, he was reacting to one or more bad experiences with New York Jews. Well, here I am: a Brooklyn-born Jew. Somehow, Joyce didn't learn about this until it was too late – she already was in love with me and I with her, a few months after meeting during our first year at Hartwick College in Oneonta, New York.

Joyce went home to Buffalo for spring break that first year of college. I was planning to drive there for a visit after a few days at home with my parents who live close to New York City. When her dad found out who she was serious about, and that I would be coming in a few days to visit, he was not pleased. Then I telephoned Joyce, and who should pick up the phone – her dad. Because I didn't know about his prejudice, I launched headlong into getting to know this special young woman's father. When it finally came time to get his daughter on the phone, he covered the mouthpiece of the phone and whispered, "Joyce, I really like this young man!"

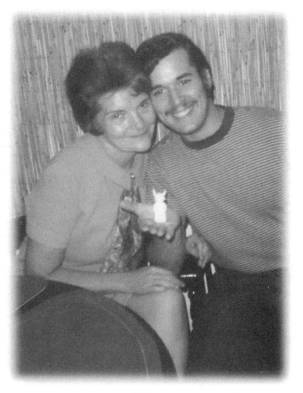

Louise and Barry in 1969.

I arrived in Buffalo on the afternoon of the first night of Passover. Joyce's mom greeted me like a long-lost friend, then asked if they could take me to the local temple for the service. I was surprised, but readily agreed. The real surprise, however, was to come that evening.

As Louise, Hank, Joyce and I walked into the temple, a continuous stream of people welcomed Louise by name. I was starting to wonder how all these people knew her, when the rabbi called out her name, quickly approached and gave her a big hug. Now I was truly stymied.

After the service, I found out the secret to Louise's fame. Before this congregation had their own temple, they met every Friday evening at the church where Louise was secretary. That explained how they all knew her, but it didn't explain how they loved her. That was her doing – her warm welcome, her friendliness, her lack of prejudice, and her sun-like smile. Now I understood. It was the same way she welcomed me into her life – and her heart.

Not that our relationship as mother and son-in-law was perfect. From time to time, we hurt each other's feelings or got angry, just like any relationship. She criticized me for not making more money. I criticized her for interfering too much in our lifestyle. But in the end we always came back to love.

She always respected that I was a doctor, even though she sometimes had trouble understanding my nontraditional approach. When our second daughter,

Mira, was born in 1981, Louise came for a visit to "help with the baby." She developed a bad cough, which progressed to severe bronchitis with fever. Not only were Joyce and I caring for a new baby, but also a very sick and bed-ridden Louise. One evening I sat on the side of her bed and gently but firmly prescribed she stop smoking. She had started smoking as a teenager, when her sister Almeda told her she would never be asked out on a date unless she started smoking. Louise looked up at me and I saw a silent resolve forming in her face. She never smoked another cigarette from that day on, and often credited her "son-in-law, the doctor" for saving her life.

Then, so many years later, she began her slow physical decline. Her body was winding down like an old clock. Her physical abilities were slowly but surely leaving her, but each seemed to be replaced by a spiritual ability. She lost bladder and bowel control, but gained a deeper ability to receive love and care from others. She lost her independence, but gained spiritual wisdom.

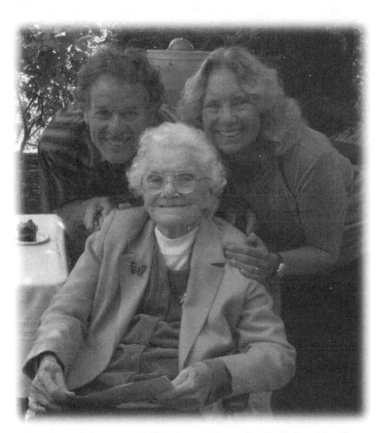

Barry and Joyce with Louise on her ninetieth (and last)
birthday party at her church, Mar 19, 2007.

I remember one time helping her walk into the
bathroom, then helping to pull down her pants and
remove her diaper. With a painful look of embarrass-

ment, she said, "Oh, Barry, here you are a man and my son-in-law, having to do all this."

I reminded her, "Grandma, remember I'm also a doctor."

"Oh, I forgot." And a look of peace came over her face.

"But that's not all, Grandma. Please remember I feel blessed to be able to give back to you all the love you've given me over the years."

With the look of a child in wonder she asked, "Really?" but the broad smile gave away her genuine joy and understanding.

She was losing some short-term memory, but her long-term memory was improving, as was her ability to live in the moment. This was an amazing gift to me as well as everyone who came into her presence. Toward the end of her life, every time she looked into my eyes, I felt bathed in love. The curtain of ego had thinned to the point where it was no longer able to block the light, just as the summer fog where we live close to the Pacific Ocean eventually dissipates, allowing the full radiance of the sun.

Experiencing Louise's passing has been truly transforming for me, my first experience of the gradual dying of a loved one. The process of sitting day by day with a slowly dying mother-in-law has allowed me to experience death in a new way. Louise's dying process was gradual enough to allow integration of every detail, every moment. Even as her bodily processes were shutting down one by one, it became clear that her soul processes did not depend on her body. The radiance of her smile increased as her bodily function decreased. The depth and peacefulness of her gaze, right up to the end, required me to completely let go of my busy thoughts so my eyes could meet hers in that utter stillness. Her clear consciousness allowed me to be present in a profound way.

In those final days, being with Louise was like being in a deep meditation. One moment, her eyes would hold me rooted in this world. The next moment, she would drift into another world, her eyes still fixed upon mine, taking me with her to an unseen place of greater love and beauty. Louise showed me the grace of dying.

Not long before she passed, Louise whispered to me, "You know, Barry, you're more than my son-in-law. I love you as a son."

With tears in my eyes, I looked into her physically fading but spiritually shining eyes and whispered back, "You know, Grandma, you used to be a mother-in-law, but now your love and acceptance of me has transformed you into a mother."

I felt moved to start singing one of my favorite songs from Cole Porter:

I give to you and you give to me,
true love, true love.
And on and on it will always be,
true love, true love.

As I sang, her feeble yet loving hands and arms reached up for me, and we kissed and hugged.

Good-bye to John-Nuri – August 16

TODAY WAS THE DAY JOHN-NURI WAS LEAVING for college. He was flying early to Lewis and Clark College in Portland, Oregon because he had been hired as a river guide for the freshman orientation trip. He would be both a freshman in orientation, as well as working as a river guide. He was excited to begin this wonderful new experience in his life. There was also the usual mix of emotions for any freshman in college as they leave behind their family and friends. But for John-Nuri there was an even greater emotional component. He knew he would never again see his beloved grandma in this lifetime.

John-Nuri and his grandma had a very special relationship. My parents moved next door to us from Buffalo when he was only three. John-Nuri spent as much time over with Grandma and Grandpa as he did with us. They had all the time in the world for him, playing Checkers, Uno, Crazy Eights, Hearts and any other game he wanted. Grandma baked cookies with him and taught him to make pies. (He is still the best pie baker in the family.) Grandma also kept her cupboards and refrigerator well stocked with food we

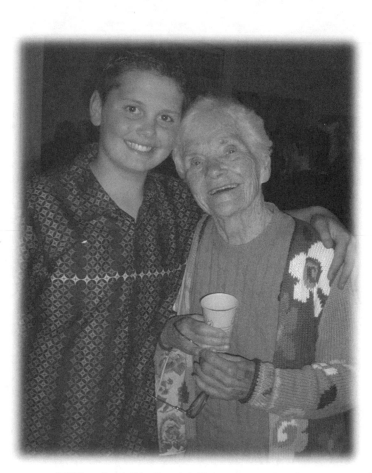

2003 – John-Nuri's eighth-grade graduation.

never bought for him, like potato chips, sugar cookies,
ice cream and cream cupcakes.

Every Saturday morning at 8am sharp, they had a
big pancake breakfast together. This was their special

time for talking. The rest of us wandered over around 9:30.

John-Nuri had five friends – Mark, Bodhi, Daniel, Roxie and Will – whose grandmas lived far away and didn't get to visit much. They all needed a grandma, so my mom adopted them all. As soon as they would come to play, their first stop was to go over to Grandma's for a cookie and her special love.

Grandma was also the matron at Mount Madonna School, the small private school John-Nuri attended. She came to every event, even when she was in a wheelchair. Sometimes everyone would stand when she would enter the room, for she was always the oldest person attending. She never missed a volleyball game, except the last year, and the boys all called her their lucky charm. Coach Patrick always ran and gave her a big hug.

My dad died when John-Nuri was ten years old. He was dearly loved and appreciated by each one of us and we missed him very much. John-Nuri took it upon himself to be my mother's protector. He started spending even more time with her. They loved to talk with one another and had a lot of private jokes. He loved to laugh at some of her favorite sayings like, "You look busier than a one-armed paper hanger" or "I haven't had this much fun in a month of Sundays." We have never had TV reception at our house and Grandma had a satellite dish, so they also enjoyed watching a few shows together on her TV.

Gradually, over the next seven years, their relationship changed. John-Nuri grew to be 6'4" and very strong and skillful in his body. She started shrinking and became more and more frail. Starting when John-Nuri was fourteen years old, he subtly began taking care of her while giving her the idea she was still taking care of him. At that time, whenever we would leave for a weekend workshop we would ask him, "Watch out for Grandma, but let her feel she is still taking care of you."

Their relationship totally changed when John-Nuri was just seventeen years old. Barry and I took a much needed weekend vacation for Father's Day. My mom was not driving at that point, so I had people coming to take her places and visit with her for much of the weekend. Her special friends, Marion and Jess, were going to take her to church that Sunday. Everything was arranged for Grandma, and John-Nuri was in charge of keeping an overall watch on things. At this point my mom was still cooking for herself, and able to do everything but drive.

Sunday morning, she got up early and was getting dressed for church, when she slipped and fell in the bathroom and couldn't get up. We had purchased one of those emergency help buttons that people wear around their necks in case they fall. She hated to wear it, and so it was not on at the time. When Marion and Jess came, she was on the floor. They could not get her up and were afraid she had hurt herself, so they called 911.

Meanwhile, John-Nuri was sound asleep after staying up late the night before. Awakened by the loud sirens of emergency vehicles coming up the driveway, he ran over to her apartment just as Grandma was being carried down the steps in a stretcher. Our oldest daughter, Rami, who also lives on our sixteen wooded acres, was not home and he couldn't contact our second daughter, Mira, who lives just fifteen minutes away. The ambulance driver told him he had to follow the ambulance and help at the hospital. Suddenly, responsibilities beyond his age were thrust upon him.

At the hospital, John-Nuri sat with Grandma. She was yelling at the nurses and doctors to let her go home and behaving in ways she never does. She has always described herself as "a child of the Depression," and she hated the way doctors ran expensive tests. She was convinced nothing was wrong with her, and she just wanted to go back to her home and get into bed. True to her fears, after six hours of tests and a bill of

$4,000, it was decided that she was only bruised and sent home.

John-Nuri sat with her and held her hand and asked her to calm down, while explaining to the nurses and doctors that his grandma must be afraid, for she never acted in other than kind ways. Finally, his sister Mira joined him at the hospital, followed by Rami, and then Barry and me, making it back from a distance of many miles. In the time he sat with her alone in the hospital, he told me he realized their relationship had now totally changed. She used to care for him and now he needed to care for her.

This day changed everything for my mom and for us. I mark this day as the beginning of her dying process. Although she was not seriously hurt, she became afraid. We could no longer leave her alone for more than an hour or two. She was no longer willing to walk by herself and would only get up or walk if we were holding her hand. She stopped doing anything for herself that involved her being on her feet, for fear of falling. Even if we were holding her hand, she was still afraid she would fall again. Since her life changed, our lives also had to change. Barry and I cut down on our work schedules. Rami and Mira agreed to help on a more regular basis. My mom moved into needing constant care.

With what little time he had, John-Nuri willingly accepted the need to help with Grandma's care. She was so proud when he took her to church each Sunday and was as happy as could be when he had time to take her to the beach. He was patient and kind with her, but also busy with all the things a high school senior has to do. Unlike other schools, Mt. Madonna senior year is the busiest of all. As my mother lost more and more of her independence, and experienced more pain in her body, Rami, Mira and John-Nuri were a constant source of joy for her.

John-Nuri was away most of the summer as a river guide and returned home one week before he was scheduled to leave for college. During that week, I wanted him to spend as much time as possible with Grandma, but of course he also had many friends he wanted to see before leaving and many fun things he wanted to do.

That's where Harry Potter helped out. When he was eight we began the series, snuggling up in bed together. Each year or two we looked forward to another one. When the last one came, we agreed to each read half by ourselves and then I would read the last half out loud to him, just like old times. In the week before he left we both sat up with Grandma and read the rest of Harry Potter. At least three hours every day we read up there in her cozy apartment. She didn't understand the book, but she couldn't care less. Just to be able to look at her precious grandson for three hours was a treat. I read and the two of them just looked at each other. John-Nuri held her hand and occasionally gave her little kisses. At that point she didn't want to talk very much, so it was perfect that she could just look at him and feel her hand in his.

In my heart I was counting down to the day John-Nuri would leave. Every parent knows both the heartache and thrill of watching their youngest child take flight and leave the nest. All week I kept painfully wondering how grandma and grandson could ever say good-bye to each other.

Finally, the day arrived. After Susie helped get Grandma ready for the day, she slept peacefully. When she awoke I told her it was now time for her to say good-bye to John-Nuri, as he would soon be leaving for college. My mother then experienced her first real resistance to her dying process.

She grabbed my hand and held tight. "No, I can't say good-bye to him. He must stay here with me. I need him. Tell him not to go."

"Mother, you know he must go."

Tears filled her eyes, "I just can't say good-bye to him. I love him too much. I'll wait here in this hospital bed until he returns again."

She has loved all her seven grandchildren equally and with an enormous amount of devotion. But perhaps because he was the youngest and she got to help raise him, John-Nuri has always held a very special place in her heart.

I took my mom's hands in mine and looked deeply into her eyes. At her request long ago, I had promised her that I would be very honest about what was happening with her body. Should I now go along with an illusion that she would still be here when he returned for Thanksgiving, or tell her the truth? I felt a deep ache in my heart as I decided to keep my promise to her and remind her of the truth.

Looking right into her beautiful tearful eyes, I told her, "Mother, you are dying. You will not be here in this body when he returns three months from now. This is your chance to really give him a gift in this final good-bye. Talk to him in a way that he will never fear death. Use the most of this time."

She continued crying and said, "I don't know if I can do that."

"You can do that, Mother, because you love him. For every hard or painful situation in my life, you have challenged me to find the gift. Now it's my turn to challenge you to find the gift in this moment and pass that onto him."

She sat for a moment in silence and dried her tears. A smile came upon her lips and she said, "I can do this. I can give John-Nuri and myself a gift right now. Please go and get him."

Fighting back my own tears, I went to get John-Nuri. He was finishing packing for his flight. I took his hands in mine and looked deeply into his eyes. "It's time to say good-bye to Grandma. Use this time wisely and don't waste words. I know you can do it."

John-Nuri took a deep breath and followed me over to Grandma's apartment. I sat in the corner and witnessed the most unbelievably beautiful scene. John-Nuri stood very close to his grandma, the oldest and the youngest in the family holding hands and looking deeply into each other's eyes.

My mom spoke first. "Wherever you are, Honey, I'll love you for your whole life. You may not know I'm there, but that's okay because I'll always love you, as I will love all my grandchildren. I'll be there for you when it's your turn to die. You can call upon my help and love any time you want."

They looked long and deep into each other's eyes. Then John-Nuri told his grandma, "I've so appreciated being able to care for you this past year."

"Honey, now I can care for you from my new home."

"Grandma, can I sing 'Every Little Breeze' one last time?"

"Please sing it, dear, but I also want you to sing it at my memorial service. And when you sing it at my service, remember I'll be singing along with you."

Although I was sitting across the room, I caught the reflection of light on a tear sliding down John-Nuri's face. There were other things spoken in that memorable good-bye, but I'd like those words to come from John-Nuri himself.

I crept quietly out of the room as John-Nuri and Grandma were saying good-bye. I was struck by the scene and wanted to stay and drink in every minute of the energy between them. John-Nuri was strong and tanned from a summer of river guiding. He was leaving home to begin an adventure at college. Grandma was white and extremely frail. She, too, was leaving to begin a journey to her new home. Her little hand in his big hand, their eyes held one another in a long and beautiful embrace. I forced myself to leave because John-Nuri had asked me to let him be alone with

Grandma. As I was leaving the room, I glanced back at my mom. Her face was radiant as she spoke to John-Nuri, "I'll be cheering you on, Honey. It's all right if you don't realize I'm there. Wherever you are, I'll be loving you and supporting you."

So This is Good-bye – John-Nuri Vissell

I ENTERED THE SOFTLY LIT ROOM.
My eyes turned immediately to my grandmother
Lying peacefully in her bed.

My mother ushered me over.
It was time to speak to my grandmother.
Unlike any other time I have spoken with her
I understood fully that this is the last time.

I was leaving for college.
I knew when I return
My grandmother would have left her body
To live in her heavenly home
In complete serenity and grace.

In this way
I attempted to construct
My final act of love towards my grandmother.

It was an intimidating prospect
To understand that in this conversation
Everything left to be expressed,
All lingering feelings and emotions towards her,

Must be said.

I tried to think of everything I wanted to say
But this was not the way it was meant to be done.

Looking into her eyes
I understood clearly what needed to be expressed.
All along I was trying to express my last emotions
To my dying grandmother
Using only words.

As I gazed into her eyes
And as she gazed into mine
I understood there was only one language
That could possibly help me express to my grand-
mother
What was in my heart...

The language of Love

And it was through this language
That I showed my grandmother
How much I loved her.

With her hand in mine
Our eyes entwined

We remained loving each other
Until one phrase
So beautiful and tender
Poured from my lips,

"I love you, Grandma."

It was enough.
It was perfect.

Leaning her head ever so softly she replied,

"I love you, too."

Then I made my last request to my dying grandmoth-
er.
I asked her to watch over me
Like her mother had done with her.

Her face lit up at my words.

Our final words had been said
But still we remained
Gazing in each other's eyes,
Loving each other.

Through My Grandma's Eyes
– John-Nuri Vissell

I WENT TO COLLEGE EARLY TO BE A RIVER GUIDE for a freshman orientation trip. Each evening, after we were off the river, I went off by myself. My grandma, one of my best friends, was dying and I would never see her again. I was out of cell phone range, so there was no way I could call. I could only imagine what was happening at home. In my stillness, I wanted to send love to her. She had taught me so much about life and now she was teaching me about death. My grandma showed no fear of death, only excitement and enthusiasm. If she could face the hardest thing in life – her death – with this positive attitude, then surely I could face any challenge with expectancy and the same enthusiasm.

My grandma also taught me about living and slowing down. Once a week I had taken her to the beach for a walk in her wheelchair. Upon arriving at Rio Del Mar Beach, I would walk around to the passenger's side and open the door for her. My grandmother would shrink away from the crisp Pacific wind into the interior of the car, making her appear even smaller than she already was.

"Ready to go?" I would say. She had lost most of her ability to walk on her own by now and for her, the prospect of getting in and out of a car was a challenging feat. It was an inspiration to see her muster up the strength to make a trip to the beach every week with me. Ten minutes and a few protests later, we would begin our short but magical jaunt along the walkway near the beach.

We were quite the spectacle, me with my six-foot-four stature, and she, bundled in blankets so tightly that the only things visible were her wizened face and wisps of white hair, tucked neatly under a worn-out pink visor. People walking by directed glances of gawking admiration, as if I were walking a queen.

The whole time I pushed her, she hardly uttered a sound, but her eyes spoke more clearly than a thousand syllables, and expressed more emotion than could have ever been derived from speech. Within my grandmother's eyes, I saw a youthful innocence and excitement that can only compare to a newborn viewing the world for the first time. Every bit of scenery, every passing man or woman was, to my grandmother, a wonderful and beautiful thing to behold. To me, it was all old news. The sand, waves, seagulls, and beach goers were something I had seen practically every day of my life, and therefore were unworthy of my full attention. However, my grandmother may have felt she would not be able to bask in the marvels of the world for much longer. She therefore devoted herself to loving and enjoying everything and everyone she saw.

My grandmother was a great teacher in the last year of her life. I was used to rushing around, not paying attention to the simple treasures that lay bountifully all around us. I had my eyes so glued to where I was going; I didn't take any time to look at where I was, or where I had come from. It was through my grandmother's quiet mentoring that I slowly learned one of the most valuable lessons in life.

During our leisurely outings to Rio Del Mar Beach, my grandmother taught me the following, and she did so without even moving from her wheelchair:

Don't move too fast.

We certainly didn't. I saw that when I rush through life, I only end up wishing I had stopped and appreciated it a little more.

She also taught me that every single person is valuable and needs to be honored. She insisted on stopping, smiling and saying "hello" to every passerby, as if they were her dear friend. People responded to her love and would stop and say hello to her.

While we made our way down the beach, she would look at everything, taking in all that was around her. There was nothing stressful about our trips to the beach. We were never in a hurry to go anywhere. And however far we went was exactly the distance we needed to go.

Once, a funny thing happened to us at the end of our beach walk. I drive a Honda Civic, personalized with stickers. It's not hard to guess that a teenager owns the car. Plus, the assorted sports gear in the back seat also suggests that I'm an active person.

I pulled up to the beach with Grandma and parked in a "handicapped" space as I needed the extra room for her wheelchair. I then carefully placed her "handicapped" sign in the window. After she got in the wheelchair, we headed off down the beach sidewalk.

When I returned forty-five minutes later my car was in the air, ready to be towed away. I wheeled my grandma up to the tow-truck driver and said, "Is there a problem, Sir?"

He looked at me, then he looked at Grandma and said, "Oh, *****!!!" He then got out and reluctantly checked for the blue handicapped placard which was still in the window where it was supposed to be. My car was lowered and a deep apology given. My grandma, who had no idea what was going on but always tried to see good in every person, took his hand

and said, "You are such a kind man for coming all the way out here just to check on my grandson's car."

At the end of our beach walks, we would return to my car, which was thankfully always still there. I would help her into her seat, put on her favorite Frank Sinatra songs, and listen to her sing along in joy and delight with a youthful smile on her face, as if she was hearing each song for the first time.

I will never forget my grandma and the unconditional love she showed me. She taught me about slowing down, seeing the good in all people, appreciating the small things in life, and not fearing death. If my grandma could be so positive about the experience of death when she was in diapers, suffering pain and helplessness, then I can find a positive attitude for the hard things that come into my life as well. Helping to care for her in those last months of her life was a gift I will never forget.

Two months after my grandma died, I was asked to sing an opera song at a music festival as a fundraiser for the music department. All of the students would be in the audience, as well as my current and future professors. I like singing a lot, but opera? It was just not my thing. Right before I was set to go on stage by myself, I peeked out and realized there must have been over a thousand people there. I felt nervous and unsure of myself. I closed my eyes and right away I could hear my grandma's voice speaking her last words to me: "Wherever you are, Honey, I will be cheering you on." How could I fail with that kind of support?

Her Angel Tells a Secret – August 17

AFTER SHE HAD HER MORNING NAP, my mother and I were sitting together mostly just looking into each other's eyes. We kept telling each other in different ways how much we loved each other. It was a sweet and precious time between us. Suddenly, my mother's eyes darted across the room and she stared at the ceiling.

"Mother, what is it?" I asked. But she could not hear me, absorbed in whatever was up at the ceiling.

After perhaps five minutes, she once again looked at me and said, "My angel came to remind me that I have just a short time left. Oh, I am enjoying this experience so much!"

In that moment I had an idea and asked, "Mom do you think it would be all right to ask your angel who Rami is going to marry?"

She brightened up and said, "That's a splendid idea. I'd sure like to know myself right now. It might take me a minute to call her."

She looked to the ceiling again and said, "Dear Angel, could you please tell me who my granddaughter is going to marry? I would really like to know before I die." There was a long silent pause, while I allowed myself to ponder Rami's situation.

Our daughter, Rami, had been engaged to a wonderful man named River. My mother absolutely adored him and treated him as if he were one of her very own grandchildren. He usually attended the Saturday morning pancake time and sometimes would stay to help her clean her refrigerator or other jobs that needed doing. He loved her very much.

The year before my mom died, Rami and River's relationship ran into difficulties that the rest of us didn't understand, and River left the relationship. He and Rami stopped talking altogether. This was a very painful time for Rami. My mother could never accept that River no longer came for pancakes and was not in Rami's life. Every so often during Saturday breakfast time she would ask hopefully if River was coming, and each time she would be told the same thing: that River and Rami were no longer together and she must accept that. Only she never could! She would always say in response, "But River would make such a good husband for you, Rami."

Two months before my mother died, I called River and asked if he would please come and visit my mother, as she wouldn't stop talking about him. He was thrilled and showed up on his motorcycle. He bounded upstairs to her apartment and warmly embraced her. They sat as close as could be on her couch while he held her hand and told her how much he loved her.

My reverie was suddenly interrupted by my mother excitedly telling me, "Joyce, my angel said that Rami will marry River!"

Oh dear, I thought. She still can't let go of that after one full year. To my mom I said, "Mother, you know that isn't going to happen."

"But Joyce, my angel told me quite certainly that Rami will marry River."

I also liked River very much and wished this were true, but all evidence pointed the other way, and I knew I needed to accept that truth for my daughter's sake. I looked at my mom and she looked so innocent, fully accepting what she had heard. But still I said, "Mom, is it possible that your angel made a mistake?"

"No," she said. "My angel was so positive and convincing."

I let the subject drop. She closed her eyes. I was about to leave the room when she suddenly opened her eyes and in an excited voice said, "Joyce, I really want River to come to my memorial service. This is very important to me!" Then she slyly smiled.

I asked her, "So what is that smile about?"

She mischievously responded, "My angel and I have a secret."

I assured her that I would invite him. She closed her eyes with the same sly smile upon her lips and drifted off to sleep.

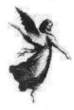

Sometime later, with Rami's permission, I invited River to Grandma's memorial service. Rami spoke at the service and I noticed that she wore extra pretty clothes and make-up. After the service, Rami and River talked for the first time in nine months. They got together that evening, and have been together ever since. Two years later, they were married in our backyard. As I was telling this story at their wedding ceremony, I could almost hear my mom's voice saying to me, "I told you River would make a good husband for Rami. See, my angel *was* right!"

Christmas in the Evening – August 17

THE HOSPICE NURSES TOLD ME THAT DEATH could come at any time in the next two weeks. I was checking on my mother more frequently. She had slept all afternoon and, in the evening, Barry and I crept over together to check on her. She was unusually still, and from a short distance we could not hear her breathing. Barry whispered to me, "Maybe this is it." We quietly and reverently moved to her bedside and put our ears very close to her mouth to see if we could hear her breathing.

Suddenly she opened her eyes and proclaimed in a triumphant voice, "Merry Christmas!!"

Barry and I jumped back, terrified. My mother was the one who was supposed to be dying, but in that moment it was our two hearts that almost stopped beating.

She asked, "Isn't it Christmas? There's so much light, surely it must be Christmas. And I see angels everywhere. There's an angel right over your heads. Don't you see her? Oh, it's so beautiful. I wish you could see it all!"

She took our hands in hers and said, "Life offers so many gifts, and the experience of dying is perhaps one of the greatest. If I just focused right now on this pain-ful old body and all that it isn't doing for me, then I would indeed be a very cranky, unhappy, old person. But I'm choosing to focus on the gift of death and so I'm able to experience the world I'm going into. It's more beautiful and wondrous than I ever could have imagined or dreamed of."

After about fifteen minutes, she squeezed our hands and said, "It's so good of you to check on me, but I think I would like to go back to the angels and the feeling of Christmas." She closed her eyes and was gone once more.

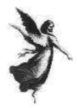

My mother always looked for the gift in every sit-uation of life. True, she was not perfect in this quest. She had trouble finding the gift when I took away her driver's license, and the one time she had to be rushed to the hospital after she fell. But in everything else that I can remember about her, eventually she was able to find a gift. She lived her life in gratitude, and therefore many people were attracted to being with her.

My mother has always challenged me to find the gift in every situation. When I was thirteen years old, my father's engineering company fell apart when his boss died. For the first time, my father was out of work. At the same time, symptoms from his childhood polio returned, and he was unable to work for four years. My mother had to support our family of four on a minimum wage church secretary job. She sat me down and told me she was going to give me ten dollars a month allowance. This was all the money that she could afford. If I needed new shoes, clothes, school supplies or anything else, I needed to take it from the ten dollars. Then she said, "You will find babysitting jobs to supplement this. I know that this is hard because you go to a school where people are very wealthy. But you will find a gift in this situation that will bless your whole life."

At the time, I didn't know how I could possibly do this. My friends all got much more allowance than ten dollars a month, as well as all the money they needed to buy new clothes and shoes. How was I going to make it? However, my mother was right. I found a gift in this four-year situation. I learned to sew all of my own clothes as well as knit my own sweaters. I also ran a highly active babysitting service, earning fifty cents an hour. I became resourceful and confident in my abilities to take charge of my own life.

When I was forty years old, we were pregnant with our third child. My parents were visiting for Christmas. My midwife came for my six month exam. After examining me, a worried look crossed her face and she told me I must go to the hospital for an ultrasound. I did not suspect anything wrong, though Barry looked concerned as well. Our two young daughters wanted to come with us and so we all went to the hospital.

At the hospital, three different ultrasound technicians examined me and quickly left the room. Finally, a doctor came into the room and rapidly did a fourth ultrasound. Without any compassion, he clumsily announced to our family, "The baby is dead." Then he quickly left, taking Barry with him.

Nothing could have prepared me for that devastating news or the way it was given to me. The girls and I were crying when Barry returned from talking to the doctor. He ushered us out of the hospital and called my parents to come and pick up our daughters so that we could go to the Ob-Gyn doctor. While we were waiting for my parents, the four of us were holding each other and crying. Mira, who was five years old at the time, had only wanted a baby sister. She looked at each of us and said, "I'll take a brother if that will help." We all had to smile at her innocence.

When my parents arrived, my mom asked to have a moment alone with me. She held me while I cried. Then she looked me into my eyes and said, "You are my daughter, Joyce, and I want you to find a gift in this situation. When my twin boys died before you were born, I thought I could never be happy again. But I knew that I must find a gift in the situation, and eventually I did. Two years after they died, you were born. God will send you another gift to replace what has been taken. You do not know the form this gift will take, but there will be a gift. Try and give thanks ahead of time for this gift, and it will help you with the pain you are feeling right now."

My grief in losing this baby was indeed very deep. I kept remembering my mother's words to me and tried to be grateful in advance for the gift that was to come, whatever that would be. Because the experience of losing the baby had been so painful to me, I had closed my mind to the possibility of another pregnancy. Two years after the death of our third child, I received a total surprise. I was pregnant with our son, who has indeed been a great gift to all of us.

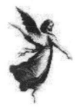

The one area where my mother had difficulty finding a gift concerned our work, especially Barry's. My mother often commented, "Barry is an MD. Why don't you have more money? Why do you have to buy clothes from the used clothing store? Why isn't Barry practicing normal medicine or psychiatry? Why don't you both stop what you are doing with these strange workshops and be a nurse again and Barry use his MD?"

The biggest source of conflict between us was when our first book, *The Shared Heart*, was published in 1984. We had been very vulnerable and honest in that book, and my mother was shocked. There was nothing in there about her, but she was embarrassed by our frankness about our own relationship. Still living in New York State at the time, she told me she hoped our book would remain a "California book."

In 1989, five months after our son John-Nuri was born, we experienced one of the biggest earthquakes in California's history, the 7.1 Loma Prieta Earthquake. The epicenter was five miles from our home. The little rented home we had lived in for thirteen years was totally and completely destroyed, along with almost everything in it. Barry and I, Rami, Mira and baby John-Nuri had all been in the house and miraculously escaped with our lives. All phone communication in Santa Cruz County was severed. Nationwide TV was showing the most horrendous shots of our community.

Back home in Buffalo, my parents were concerned and, as the death toll mounted, they feared for our lives. They looked on the map and realized that our home was very close to the epicenter. It took five very difficult days before they knew we were alive. During that time, people from all over the country were calling them to find out about us. My mother's name and city had been mentioned in our second book, *Models of Love*. People who read that book found out my parents' number and called. My mother told me that many people called her each day. In the course of the calls, they told her how much our work and books had helped their lives.

Finally, after five days, my parents were able to get through to us. I cried as soon as I heard my mother's voice. I had been strong until then, keeping it together for the children and trying to move the few remaining unbroken things somewhere else. But hearing my mother's voice broke all my reserves of strength, and I felt like a little girl needing comfort. She did not sympathize with me over broken treasures or being homeless. She told me in no uncertain terms I needed to focus on gratitude and the gift that we were all alive. That was just like my mother to focus on what was most important in times of crisis. She also told me about all the phone calls from people who had read our books and taken our workshops.

Then she said words I had needed for many years. "Joyce, I never understood what your books and work were about. I thought you should both use your medical training to help people. All of these many people who called told me how important your work is in their lives. Now I understand you are a doctor and nurse of the soul. From now on I am going to totally support you in your work. This understanding has been the gift of these very difficult five days of not knowing if you, Barry or the children were alive."

My mother really used this gift of understanding and went on to become our greatest supporter and fan. Whenever we had a workshop in our home, she made cookies and coffee and left a note on our door to welcome people and suggest they come up to her house for some refreshments. Those who went were served her famous cookies, and they received a bonus – her love. She also made sure to tell everyone how fortunate they were to be able to do a workshop with us. Everyone loved my mother, and many people who came for workshops also went up to visit her during the breaks. Most people coming down from her apartment usually said, "Wow, your mom sure does support your work!"

Every single day my mother lay dying she looked at me and said, "I'll be helping you with your work from my new home. You'll know I'm there and people will feel my love." The very last words my mother spoke directly to me were, "Remember: I'll never leave you, and I'll help you with your work."

Final Message to Bruce's Family
– August 18

MY BROTHER BRUCE AND HIS WIFE RUTH live in Minnesota. They have four grown children, two of them married, and three grandchildren. My mother adores each and every one. Usually she spends a part of each summer with my brother's family. This summer, it would have been impossible for her to go.

My brother gathered his entire family in his living room and told them they were going to call Grandma, and this would be the last time they would hear her voice. As a family they practiced singing her favorite hymn, "How Great Thou Art."

When my brother called, Barry picked up the phone. My brother is a Ph.D. electrical engineer, and he loves technology. He and Barry have often bonded over technology, and this was no different. They spent quite a while figuring out the best speaker system so that his whole family could hear the conversation with Grandma, as well as Barry, my mom, and me. While there were multiple calls going back and forth, I told my mother that Bruce and his whole family were on the phone to sing to her.

Her attachment to these loved ones was so strong that she stepped out of her dying process for the second time. She said, "I'll tell them I'll come and stay with them next summer. I really want to see them all again."

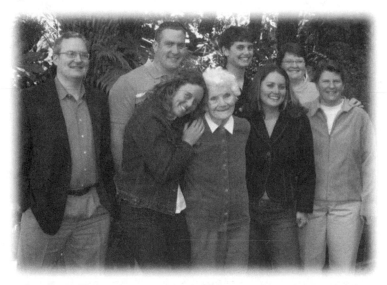

Louise with her seven grandchildren on her eighty-eighth birthday. From left: Allen, Aaron, Rami, John-Nuri, Mira, Amy, and Anne.

As was the case when she was saying good-bye to John-Nuri, I knew that I must be honest and live up to my promise to her. Again I took a deep breath and inwardly asked for help. Taking her hands in mine, I gently spoke to her, "Mother, you are dying. This is the last time they will hear your voice. Say something they will always remember."

A look of sadness crossed her face as she said, "Oh, I forgot I'm dying. I really don't want to die now that they have called. I want to go and visit them."

Once again, I had to summon my courage to speak the truth. "Mother, you know that's impossible. This is the last time they will hear your voice. What do you most want to say to them?"

She was thoughtful for a moment, then a smile crossed her face as she said, "Thank you for reminding me of what is most important. I got lost in my desire to be with them. Now I know what to say."

Finally the two men figured out the best speaker-phone setup, and it was time to sing to Grandma. My brother's family sang her favorite hymn and then took turns telling her how much they loved her. When it was time for my mom to speak, she said, "I love you all so much, and I'll always be with you in your heart. I won't need a phone from now on to call you. You'll hear me in your heart. I'll call you often."

Barry and I had tears in our eyes from the beauty of the message. My brother later called and told me that each of his family, even the active seven and nine-year-old grandsons, had tears in their eyes upon hearing Grandma's last message to them.

After they hung up, my mom had a look of total satisfaction upon her face as she said, "Joyce, thank you so much for reminding me that I am dying. I probably would have just gone on and on about wanting to come and see them next summer. That might have made them very sad, for they know I can't come. Now I feel I said just the perfect thing for them to remember me by."

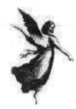

I feel very thankful for the harmony that existed between my brother and me during the last months and especially the last three weeks of my mother's life. In our work we often hear stories of horrendous situations that occur between siblings around the death of their parent. If I could put a percentage upon it, I would say that fifty percent of the cases where a parent is dying there is tension and fighting between siblings around the care of their parent. People assume that everyone will come together in a peaceful, harmonious way when their parent dies but, trust me, from the many stories we have heard in our work, this is often not the case.

A friend of ours reported that his two brothers fought so much over the care of their father that they were actually still fighting in the same room while the dad was taking his final breath. Our friend was the only one really present for his father's death.

Another family did not want their brother's girlfriend to be present in the room while their father was dying. They argued that she wasn't married into the family and therefore she should not be there. The brother argued that she had been the one to help him care for their father the most in the months leading up to his death. The other siblings argued so much over this that in the end the girlfriend, one of the father's main supporters and caregivers, was not allowed to be in the room.

Another family had a sibling who did not believe in Hospice. She was not involved in her mother's care in the months leading up to her death because she was a busy executive, but flew out from a distant city to be there for the final days of her mother's life. When she arrived and saw her mother in a weakened state, she insisted on terminating Hospice and taking her mother to the hospital. A big fight ensued and the poor mother's request to be in her own home was not honored as the daughter took her to the hospital.

When adult children are not prepared for the death of a parent, all kinds of unresolved feelings can come up. If a child has ignored their parent, they might feel guilty and want to make it up to them in the final days, like the case of the executive daughter. They sometimes try and shove aside other siblings that have always been there for the parent. Also, if they are close to the dying parent but have never gotten along with a certain sibling, these differences can often be magnified when they are trying to cooperate around the care of the parent.

We have also heard of several situations where one sibling will not want too much money spent on a dying parent so they can preserve their inheritance. Even though this is money that the parent has earned and saved, they do not want it spent on "frivolous" things like good home health care in the months leading up to the death.

Then there are situations where the siblings fought over how the inheritance will be handled while they were in the same room with the dying parent. These and other scenarios can be a nightmare for the dying person as well as any sibling that sincerely wants to give his or her parent a loving environment in which to die.

Since my mother's parents both died suddenly when she was fairly young, it was important for her to prepare my brother and me for her death. Ten years before she died, we both received a typed letter (on her manual typewriter) and were told to save the letter until she was dying. In this letter, she outlined exactly what she wanted for her death as well as her memorial service. We never had to guess or work it out between us. She didn't want to go to the hospital, and she didn't want to take drugs or have anything extra done to save her life when her time came. She told us she had already driven herself and gotten the legal forms for "Do Not Resuscitate." She said, "Joyce and Bruce, I want you to be happy for me when it is my time to die. I am excited and very much at peace about this process."

My brother and I are very different in so many ways, and yet we each honored how the other one cared for and loved our parents. I wanted to be there one hundred percent in my mom's care in the last eight years after my dad died. My brother was content to have her come for a long visit in the summer. Three years before she died, he took her on a trip that she treasured and talked about constantly. He traveled with her to the tiny town of Westville, Pennsylvania, where she had spent her childhood. They visited the grave sites of her parents and spent a week walking the little town and talking to people. They actually met a man older than my mom who remembered her Swedish family with the eight children. They sat and talked with him the rest of the day. They visited the house in which my mother was born and where her mother's open casket lay in the living room for one week before being placed in the ground.

I would not have taken my mother on that long trip or been interested in those things, but my brother used a week of his vacation to do that for her. He also came by himself for two weeks in the last two months of my mother's life, when we had to be away working. I had hired a woman to do all of the things that I do, but he sat with Mom and talked, and she loved it.

If I could pass on wisdom to anyone whose parent is still alive, start talking to your siblings about what will happen when your parent dies. It is better to begin this process while your parent is still healthy and active.

Some worthwhile advice to any parent: when your children are grown and the time feels right, start preparing them for your death. If you don't feel comfortable talking to them about it, then write a letter and ask them to keep it until the time arrives. I will always be grateful for the letter that my mother sent us and for the agreement that passed between my brother and I concerning her care. I have known quite a few siblings that fought so much during the time of their parent's death that they were never able to be close again. My brother and I are very close. In fact, our mother's dying process has brought us even closer.

Communion Afternoon – August 18

LATER THAT SAME DAY, her wonderful minister Bob Bowles and his wife Margie finally came back from their summer vacation in Greece. They immediately came over to see Grandma and brought communion for her. To say my mom loves Bob Bowles would be an understatement. She adores him! It would seem the sun rises and sets around her wonderful minister. She talked about him so much that our family sometimes would challenge her to go five minutes without bringing up his name. She couldn't do it. She never says Bob. It is always Bob Bowles. One of Rami's friends, who is a talented cartoonist, made a picture of a man with the name Bob on his shirt bowling at a bowling alley. The cartoon was titled, "Bob Bowles." My mom loved the cartoon so much she had it framed and put it right next to her bed. Of course, everyone who came to see her had to see the cartoon, and then hear all about Bob Bowles. In the last weeks of her life, she had us place a framed picture of her and Bob right in the bed with her. This picture rested right next to a picture of my dad. She spent hours looking at the two pictures.

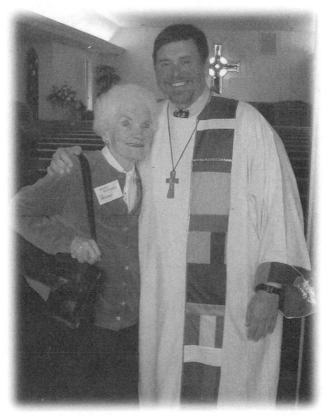
Louise with her beloved minister, Bob Bowles

Bob and Margie walked into her apartment, and my mother's smile and radiance could have brought light to a darkened room. Bob led us all in a beautiful communion service.

As he was preparing to leave, he asked my mom what she would most want at her memorial service.

Without hesitating, she replied, "I want my grandson, John-Nuri, to sing my Louise song." Then she sang a little of the song, "Every little breeze seems to whisper Louise. Birds in the trees seem to whisper Louise. Can it be true, someone like you could love me, Louise?"

Bob smiled but firmly said, "Louise, you know we don't allow songs like that in our church." He runs a very traditional church service.

"But Bob," she said with a disarming sweetness, "That's the only thing I want, and you asked me what I most want."

I watched the conflict in his face. He clearly loved my mother, yet he was the minister of a conservative church of mostly older people.

He breathed a deep sigh of resignation to the wishes of a dying elder – in fact, one of the first female elders of the Presbyterian Church in America. "All right, Louise, he can sing your favorite song at your memorial."

My mom smiled brightly. "I'm so happy. I told him I would be singing right along with him."

Bob and Margie kissed my mom and wiped their tears as they reluctantly left the room. My mom looked completely happy as she said, "What a wonderful day. I'm going to go to sleep now." She slept until the next morning.

Last Day for Visitors – August 19

THIS SUNNY SUNDAY MORNING, I had a series of visitors come to see my mother. She sat up in her bed, her face aglow with joy to be seeing everyone. It was just like her to be the life of the party, telling jokes and laughing. She was so alive and engaging that none of us could have suspected that she would die in just one week. Typical of my mother, she appreciated each and every person. She always had an encouraging word to share. Each person knew that they had a very safe and special place within her heart.

The last visitors were seven women from her church. The main soloist was there and sang Mom's favorite hymn, "How Great Thou Art." The other ladies then led her in the entire church service. At the end they all said prayers for her journey. Some of the women there were almost as old as she was. It was very touching to witness the love and caring they have for my mom. At the end she told them, "You are my family. Sunday was my favorite day because I got to see you each week. Thank you for all of your love. I'll be waiting for you when you take this great journey. Always know how much I love you."

As they were saying good-bye, all of these women knew they would never see my mother again. But there were no tears or sorrow. My mother was so upbeat that it was contagious. The ladies said good-bye to her the way one would say good-bye to someone who is going on a much-dreamed-of vacation.

By 1PM, all the visitors had left. My mother looked tired, but deeply satisfied, as she said, "I loved my visitors so much. This was all so special. But please no more visitors. I need to concentrate and get ready for my special journey. It's now taking too much energy to be in this world with visitors. I need to be in my other world." She closed her eyes and didn't open them again until the next morning. I can only imagine all that she was experiencing during that time.

I stayed with my mother for a while longer watching her sleep. Now that she no longer wanted visitors, I knew she was truly getting ready to leave this world.

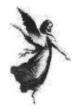

VISSELL

To say that my mother was quite possibly the friendliest person anyone had ever known was not an exaggeration. It was the truth.

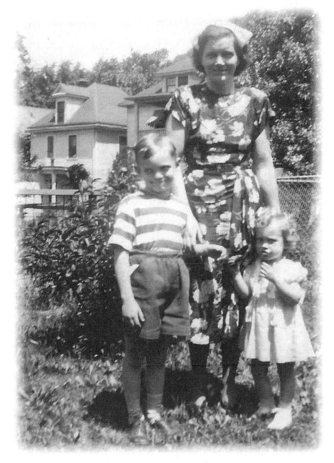

Louise with Bruce and Joyce.

When my brother and I were growing up, we used to groan when she would stop the car for what she said was just a tiny errand. No errand was small for my mother. Wherever she went, she inevitably saw a friend of hers and took the time for conversation. If she met a person one time and talked to them, then that person became a friend and she enthusiastically greeted them forever more. Everyone loved my mother.

When she was able, she drove the seven minutes from our property and walked on the Rio del Mar Beach sidewalk every day for one mile. At the entrance to the walk, there used to be a group of guys over fifty who sat on the narrow wall leading to the sidewalk. Several of these men were homeless. At first when I would bike by them on my frequent bike rides, I felt a little afraid if no one else was around. They always tried to engage me in conversation, but I just biked on by. Well, my mother stopped to talk to them on her walks and, before you knew it, she was sitting on the wall with them.

Her favorite was a man named Pat who lived in his old beaten-down motor home in the parking lot. Pat was a large man, poorly dressed, with missing teeth. My mother thought he was just the nicest man. Every day she went to the beach hoping to be able to sit on the wall with Pat. I got to know all of these men through my mom.

One day, when she was perhaps eighty-seven years old, she was sitting on the wall with the group of men laughing and having a grand time when a number of ladies from her church came walking by. They were shocked to see that Louise was associating with *these* men. My mom tried to introduce them, but the ladies walked on by. They called her that night and told her she should be more careful. She responded that they were children of God, too, and deserved her love. Pat made my mother an official member of the "Wall Sitter's Club," and she felt very honored.

In their retirement, my parents participated in feeding the homeless every week. My mother usually made her famous old-fashioned fruit-filled jello and brought it to the church. Most of the people would simply drop off their food and leave. Not my parents. They stayed and sat with the men and treated them with as much respect as if they were at the White House for a dignitary's dinner. They knew all of the mens' names and sincerely cared about their well-being. After my dad died, my mother continued this weekly tradition until she was eighty-nine. She often said that those men were some of her closest friends. It makes me think of Jesus' statement: *"What you do to the least of God's creatures, you do to me."*

I remember clearly a time when I was twelve years old. It was a cold Saturday morning and I was up in my room playing by myself. My mother came in and asked why I didn't have a friend come over and play with me. I answered, "I really don't have good friends that would want to come to my house and play with me."

In no uncertain terms she replied, "Joyce, in order to have a friend you must BE a friend. Concentrate on how you can BE a friend to others and, before you know it, you will have lots of friends."

I have never forgotten that time or her words to me. Because of that advice, I treasure the friends that I have and always try to BE a good friend.

My Grandma, My friend – Mira Vissell

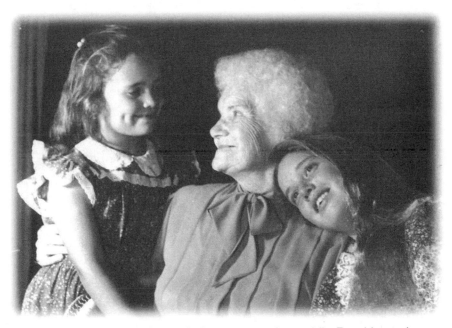

Mira and her grandma adoring one another, while Rami leans in happily. – photo by Carla Annette

MY GRANDMA WAS A TRUE FRIEND TO ME. No matter what was going on in my life, I knew that Grandma loved me unconditionally. She believed I could do anything I put my heart into and was very proud of me. I loved to bring my school papers over to her when I was younger. She would sit right down, read them carefully, and comment on different points I was trying to make. She always had something positive to say about my work.

When I was living at home and my parents went away for weekend workshops once or sometimes twice a month, my grandma made delicious meals for us. She would set the table with bright paper napkins so that it seemed like a party. She would make a special dessert for us – a cake, cookies, or her special jello and fruit dish served with whipped cream. Even though I was on a school volleyball team that seemed to lose each match, Grandma came to each game and cheered me on like it was the Olympics.

She was such a special friend to me for my whole life that when I was twenty-five years old and my mother asked if I would help care for her in her last year, I knew I wanted to say yes. I was privileged to care for her three mornings a week, and Rami took the rest. My mother, with help from my dad, did all of the afternoons and evenings.

I would arrive at my parent's house early in the morning and walk up the flight of stairs leading to my grandma's apartment next door. When I would peek in on her, she would usually still be asleep, but sometimes I would walk in and see her bright blue eyes waiting for me. A look of love and recognition would cross her face.

"Good morning, Grandma, how are you doing?" I would ask.

"Oh, good morning, Mira," she would respond.

"Today is going to be a good day, Grandma. We're going to Elder Day!!"

I would then put on a CD of her favorite music, and we would begin getting her ready. My first job was picking out a really nice outfit for her. Grandma always had dressed nicely, even if she was just going to be sitting at home for the day. In the last year of her life she didn't seem to care that much, but still we dressed her up each and every day.

The hardest part of the morning was getting her out of bed, legs first, then getting her to muster up the energy to stand up. Often this would take a few minutes of serious coaxing and reminders of what the day could offer if she ventured out of the bed. Usually she would say, "Oh, Mira, let's just skip it today." Grandma would have spent the whole day in bed if we let her. But we all knew that would lead to painful bedsores, muscle deterioration, and a host of other problems. We got her out of bed each day until the last two weeks of her life. Once on her feet, though, she would be one-pointed towards the bathroom. Helping her out in the bathroom was sometimes a struggle but sometimes she would say to me:

"Mira, you're doing a good job. You would make a good nurse."

I had been dealing with a change of careers and a change of heart from my current work. I have a college degree in Information Systems Management and realized I didn't want to do that the rest of my life. I had been thinking about the possibility of going back to school and working towards becoming a nurse. But I doubted if I had it in me to care for someone. It was during these early times of working with my grandma that I decided I really love taking care of someone.

"Grandma," I got to respond one day in the bathroom, "I'm going to study to be a nurse."

Grandma lit up and said, "I know you're going to be a great nurse. I'm so happy."

After the bathroom, we headed over to the living room for breakfast on the couch (she called it a "davenport"). She would sit and think while I quickly got her pills ready and started the oatmeal. Taking her medicines and supplements took a while. Sometimes, I would be done with the oatmeal and ready for the next step but she would still be taking the pills, one at a time. If I had anything to tell her, or a story to share, she would stop everything to listen to me. She would listen with her full attention and devotion, something that can be hard to find these days. If we were in a rush at all, I had to keep quiet during the oatmeal and pills process.

The next step of the day involved getting down the stairs to my car. Grandma would often resist, so I had to muster extra enthusiasm to convince her of what a great day lay outside her apartment. I'd bundle her up, even if it was hot outside for me. Then we would tackle the stairs, one at a time, no rush on a matter like this.

Once in my car, I would put my "Grandma List" on my iPod and away we would go. The list of music had about ten songs I had found that I knew she liked. That's all I had, so every single time in the car it was the same list of songs in the same order. But it didn't matter because when each song came on, she would belt out her accompaniment in a surprisingly loud voice. Patsy Cline, Ella Fitzgerald, Frank Sinatra, Dean Martin, Billie Holiday... they would start her singing along. It didn't matter how off-key she was, her singing would be so infectious I couldn't help but join in.

One of my three mornings, I took Grandma for a walk on the beach. Then we did her favorite thing, which was going to Deluxe Foods, a grocery store that she had been going to for fifteen years. Everyone knew her and would call out her name, as if they were greeting a beloved friend. I would push her in her wheelchair and she would pick out the food she wanted, which was mostly cookies. I made her get some healthy things as well.

She went to Elder Day two mornings a week, which was about twenty-five minutes away. Elder Day is a place where elderly people can go and hang out together and have a good time. The people in charge are nurses and very caring aides who facilitate activities for the elderly. They would play bingo, hear songs played on the piano, draw pictures, make crafts, and play games that got them to exercise.

There was a special van that would pick up the elderly at their homes and transport them and their wheelchairs, canes, and walkers back to Elder Day. I think Grandma was one of the only ones who was lucky enough to have someone drive her there personally. When we arrived, I would wheel her in. Everyone knew my grandma. The aides, nurses and other workers would all smile or say hello as we passed by. Once inside, her friends would brighten to see her.

I felt like we were getting the royal treatment. Everyone loved Grandma. She treated everyone like a special friend. I would wheel her straight up to her table which she shared with eight other very elderly people.

As soon as Grandma arrived at her table, it seemed as if a party would begin. She would say a kind word to each of the eight other people, and they would brighten with her love and caring.

As I would leave her there, the piano would be playing and the smell of coffee would drift by. I knew she would have a good time socializing and doing the different activities. I always felt so grateful for the time I would get to spend with my grandma. She enjoyed the simple pleasures of that time: singing, eating, smiling, and listening to stories.

Driving away, I turned on my iPod and Dean Martin started singing, "You're nobody till somebody loves you…" I could have changed it to my own musical favorites, but for some reason I started singing along with Dean. Computers to nursing? Could the message of this song have anything to do with my career change?

I am so grateful that I got to spend those mornings with my grandma in the last year of her life. Grandma taught me the true meaning of the word "friend." She showed me that even though a person is failing in their body and can't do much for themselves, they can still be a friend to others, offering kindness, thankfulness and appreciation. Grandma never wasted time complaining about her aches and pains like so many elderly people do. Instead, she used that energy to reach out to people and appreciate them. I think that is why so many people wanted to be around her. I know that my life has been blessed by her love and positive attitude, and I have seen many other lives blessed in the same way by her friendship.

We Are Never Alone – August 20

TODAY MY MOTHER WAS STARTED ON MORPHINE for the growing pain she was experiencing. She did not want to be on any pain medication, wanting instead to fully experience her dying process. However, the pain had increased to the point that her Hospice home health aide, Susie, could no longer do all the things that make her more comfortable, like bathe her, change the sheets, put dressings on the bed sores and all the many other things this sweet angel does for my mother. We decided that very early in the morning she would receive the smallest morphine dose possible. The nurse assured me that after five hours the drug will have totally left her system. She said that this small dose is just a little stronger than an over-the-counter pain killer. She was given the dose each morning at 6:30 and then she usually slept until two or three in the afternoon, when the drug had fully left her body.

The morphine allowed Susie to clean and change her and even wash her hair. She put on a clean white shirt and arranged her hair in little curls all over her head. She looked beautiful. After her bed bath she slept for the rest of the morning and some of the afternoon. I sat next to her, notebook in hand, trying to always be ready to write down whatever she said.

Sometime in the afternoon, I was just dozing off on the couch when she excitedly remarked, "I'm so happy to be finally joining you, Hank, in your new home. Please tell me all about it." There were long silences broken by words such as, "Oh, that is so wonderful. Wow, that must be so special. I have never experienced that before. Oh, Hank, I can't wait."

Then she started filling him in on all her activities in the eight years since he had gone. At one point she said, "Did you know that our granddaughter, Ann, had a baby girl named Emily?"

There was a silence, during which my dad must have been talking to her.

Then she said, "How do you know that she likes to wear pink all the time and sings to herself a lot?"

Pause.

"Oh, so you've seen her quite a bit. Did you know that our grandson Aaron got married?"

Pause.

"Oh, so you were there too?"

Pause.

"So you've seen everything that's happened to me. I guess there's nothing new to tell you then. Tell me more of the new home I am going to." She lay with her eyes closed.

My dad must have had a lot to say for there was a long period of silence. Every once in a while a big smile would spread across her face, so I knew he must have been telling her good things. To pass the time, I got up and went into another room and brought back some of the albums that were filled with photos that my dad took.

My dad was an avid hobby photographer. He photographed everything for memory's sake. He had photos of every inch of the family home he and my mom lived in for thirty-five years. Each bathroom was photographed from several angles, each closet, each room and even the basement, from multiple perspectives. My dad was on hand with his camera for every family event. We often teased him about the quantity of photos he took, but he kept on taking them until the day before he died. There were volumes of photos, and none of us ever studied them the way he wished we would. We would look at them several times, but he always hoped we would look at them many more times.

While my mom was lying silently with her eyes closed the entire time, I looked at the photos for quite some time, then put them back in the bedroom. I returned to the couch and sat quietly, just looking at my mom, still with her eyes closed. She suddenly startled me by saying in a loud clear voice, "Joyce, your dad's really happy you were looking at his photos."

When she spoke, I realized more deeply that I was with *both* of my parents. My dad had left his body years before, but he had never left me or his family. He was still present in my life. I knew that my mother would also never leave me. There would be no need to feel like an orphan after both of my parents have passed on. Just as my dad was present in the room, happily watching me look at his photos, so they both would be present with me throughout my life. I feel them right now as I sit at my computer writing this. They are teaching me about the enduring quality of love. They want me to know that we are never alone. True love and connection never dies; it just changes form.

Tears started flowing from my eyes as I fully comprehended that I would always have the love of my parents. Right on cue, my mother opened her eyes and looked at me with a penetrating gaze saying, "Remember, I will never leave you. Your dad and I will always be present in your life, loving and protecting you. I'm also going to help you in your work. You'll always know when I am there."

She closed her eyes again. After a while, as it was getting late, I crept out of her apartment, quietly saying, "Good night, Mom. Good night, Dad."

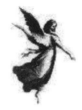

Hospice was now taking care of every detail of my mother's dying process. Susie was an enormous caring support. She showed me how to do everything for my mother, and made it easy for me. She came five mornings a week now and on the weekends another woman came and did the same. Emily, her chaplain, made regular visits several times a week. She was trained to be a comfort to all people regardless of type or lack of religion. Lara, her social worker, was a support for both my mother and for me, encouraging especially me to share my feelings. And Carol, her nurse, attended to every single detail, and instructed Susie to carry them out. There was not one second in which I felt that my mother was being neglected by Hospice in their care of her.

Everything was done to make her feel comfortable. She was in a hospital bed that could be raised either by the head or the feet. She lay upon a mechanical mattress device that gave relief to the growing number of pressure sores on her back. She even had a little tent structure that was over her feet, to ward off pressure sores on her toes from the weight of her blanket. I trained for nursing at one of the country's finest teaching hospitals, New York's Columbia University Hospital. That hospital set the bar of quality care for me. However, I must say that the care my mother received from Hospice went above and beyond even that level. And all of this care was covered by her Medicare insurance.

One of the few requirements of us as a family was to turn her every two hours. She hated this so much that we usually skipped the process to every three hours, and did not do it during the night. We would approach her bedside and, with the most enthusiasm we could muster, say, "Time to turn you."

She would look at us and plead, "Oh, couldn't you just skip it this once. I'll never tell Carol." Or, "Let's not do that. I'm dying anyway. What difference does it make?"

According to Carol and Susie, it made a big difference in her overall comfort and well-being and so reluctantly we did it. Susie had the extra sheets all arranged so that anyone could easily roll her to her other side and place a pillow there.

Throughout ninety-eight percent of my mother's dying experience, she lay with a sweet, loving smile upon her lips. But the other two percent was anything but. It was during these times of rolling her to her other side that her pain angrily said things like, "You are a mean and ungrateful daughter!"

Or to Barry, "Barry, you're supposed to be a doctor, and here you are torturing and killing me."

Or to Rami or Mira, "How could I have such an awful granddaughter to cause me so much pain?"

At first when these explosions happened I would be very upset. How could my loving Swedish mother say something like that? But then I noticed that as soon as she was turned and comfortable again, she would return to her sweet self. At first I questioned her, "Mother, why did you say that to me?"

She would look totally innocent as she asked, "What did I say?" She never could remember saying anything. When I would tell her, she would tell me that it was the pain speaking. She maintained that she could never say anything like that. Once she even struck out at Rami as she was trying to change her adult diaper. She never remembered trying to hit Rami.

As a nursing student I witnessed hundreds of births in my training. These were people from some of the poorest sections of New York City. Some were too young and ill-prepared to give birth. In the intensity of labor they would scream out, "Take this horrid thing away from me, I never want to see it." And yet these same women who wanted to kill their babies moments before, soon reached with love and affection to hold their newborn. I learned from that experience that pain definitely has its own voice, and does not necessarily reflect the true feelings of the person.

I will be forever grateful to Hospice for the loving care they provided for my mother. Without their help, it would have been almost impossible for Barry, Rami, Mira and me to provide her with what she needed to have her beautiful – and natural – dying experience.

Night Visitor – August 21

I WOKE IN THE MIDDLE OF THE NIGHT and felt I must check on my mom immediately. I crept over to her apartment. As I was walking up the stairs, from the open window I heard her talking to someone. I got a little nervous. Did someone come in the middle of the night? I sighed in relief as I stepped into the room and found only my mother in her hospital bed.

"Mom, who have you have been talking to?"

"Oh, my dear friend Thelma is here with me. She looks beautiful. She's standing right next to you now."

Thelma was my mother's very best friend at church. They always sat next to each other in church. They would wait for the other and walk in together. They also called each other several times a day. It was a big loss to my mom when Thelma died three years ago. She had many other friends at church to sit with, but no one else called to talk several times a day. And yes, on more than one occasion they got teased for their names, Thelma and Louise, a film about a pair of infamous women who went wild and disrupted several macho men's worlds.

My mother was absolutely radiant as she reported to me, evidently aware that I couldn't see her best friend, "Thelma is here to tell me about the new church she attends. She's going to hold my hand and take me there. We'll sit together again in church. She said I'll love this new church. It's very inspiring and, well, just unbelievably beautiful."

She went on to tell me that Thelma looks years younger, and very happy. I sat with my mom for a while. Thelma must have left because she went back into a deep sleep. I walked back to our house and slipped into bed, pondering my mom's night visitor.

The Invisible Surprise Party
– August 21

THIS WAS THE DATE EIGHT YEARS AGO that my dad died. My mother and I have always honored this day in some way. The first few years after he died, we would gather in the back yard by the flowering plum tree where his ashes had been placed. In later years, we simply sat together and looked at pictures of my dad. Whatever we did, the day was always honored and special. My mother often spoke of her feelings about death, but especially each year on this day she would say something like, "Remember, Joyce, death is a great adventure in life. It's something to be excited about, not dreaded. Don't be afraid of this wonderful journey our Creator has planned for us."

When I walked in at 6:30 to be with my mom for the morning, she was alert and looking at me with steady eyes.

"Do you know what day this is, Mom?"

"I sure do. This is the day that Dad died. This is the day I want to die, too."

"Well, Mother, it doesn't look like this is the day, but we can make this day special in other ways."

"I want this day to be the most special of all," she said with a smile.

When our Hospice angel, Susie, came at 7:30, we told her this was a special day. Susie got my mom all cleaned up and put on her favorite shirt, one that Dad had bought for her right before he died. She also "washed" her hair, using a special shampoo that you put on while the patient lies in bed, then can be combed out, all without water. I didn't believe it could work until I watched her. Susie used to be a hairdresser, so she made my mom's hair extra pretty. She even put lipstick on her lips and showed her how pretty she looked. My mom's response, "Not bad!"

The hour Susie spent on my mom completely tired her out, and she then slept for at least five hours. I checked on her often and she was in a very deep sleep.

Around 2:30 in the afternoon, I started climbing the steps to her apartment next door and, from the open window, it sounded as if there was a party going on, but the only voice I heard was my mom's.

"Thank you so much for coming.

Oh, it's so lovely to see you again.

It's so crowded in here, do you have enough room?

What a wonderful surprise party this is."

I turned around to look at the driveway, assuming that a crowd of visitors must have come from her church. But there were no extra cars. With a growing curiosity, I climbed the stairs and opened the door to her apartment, fully expecting a room full of people who have come to visit. Imagine my surprise to see an empty room and my mom with eyes fully opened talking and laughing with people I cannot see.

"Oh, Joyce, come in. Isn't it just so wonderful! My whole family came to visit me. Isn't my mother beautiful? I haven't seen her since she died when I was only six years old. She looks just like I remember her. And there's my dad. He's standing right next to you. I haven't seen him since I was sixteen."

I sat down on the couch. I wanted to fully experience what was happening, though I was only aware of my mom talking and laughing to people I couldn't see or hear. Though I had never met my mom's parents, I have heard stories about them for my entire life. And now they were in the room! It was like my mother inhabited two worlds at the same time, one with me in it and another with her deceased family members. I sat as quietly as I could, notebook and pen in hand, wanting to absorb this incredible experience and remember it always.

My mother is the last of eight children to die. She loved her family of origin and they were always a huge part of her life. Except for her brother, Al, who moved to California, and her brother, Carl, who died when my mother was pregnant with me, all the rest lived within a few miles of each other in Buffalo, New York. My growing-up years were spent surrounded by my aunts and cousins.

As I sat on the couch contemplating all that was happening around me, my mother continued with her party. She could see both me and relatives that I

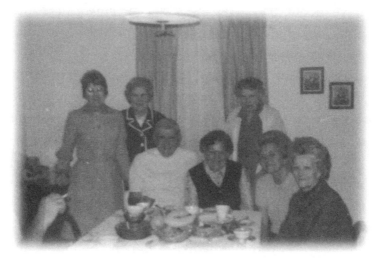

Louise and six of her siblings (from left): Betty, Gert, Al, Arlene, Dora, Louise, and Almeda.

couldn't see. I sat very quiet and alert. Surely this was an important event, a grand family reunion.

"Mom, please tell me who you are seeing."

"My whole family is here and they're waiting for me. It's so crowded. Oh, there is Sylvia. She looks so young and beautiful. She is right with Lou (her husband and my dad's older brother) and, yes, there is Paul (one of her twin sons who died a few years ago). They look great and seem so happy. Oh, Almeda (her sister) is looking so beautiful now, and there are Gert and Dora (two other sisters who never married), both looking so wonderful. There is Arlene (another sister) with John and they seem so happy and beautiful. Al and Gen look so young and beautiful. Oh, look at how special Betty (her youngest sister) looks! My mom and dad are so happy and just can't wait for me to come and join the family again."

Curious, I asked, "Mom, what about Dad? Is he here with you, too?"

"Of course Dad's here. He's been here the whole time, right next to me," she says matter-of-factly as she points to the side. "Can't you see him? He's here as clear as could be. Oh, I wish you could see Dad and my family. They are all so happy and look so beautiful. All the wrinkles are gone, all the sickness, all the problems. They look the way they did when they were young.

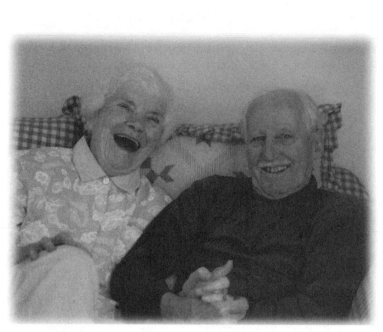

Hank always knew how to make Louise laugh.
– photo by Cindy Lou Rowe

I'm the only one here still with my wrinkles. They're so happy I'm coming back to them. After all these years, our family will be together again." Tears were flowing down my mother's cheeks as well as mine.

My mother continued enjoying her party. Then her smiling face became serious as she looked towards the door and said, "Bill, what are you doing here? Where is Esther? I'm happy to see you. I'm just surprised."

I wondered who Bill was. We didn't have a relative named Bill. The mystery of this visitor was cleared up the following Christmas *after* my mom died. She received several cards from people we were unable to notify of her passing. One of these cards was from Esther, who explained that Bill, her husband, had died in May of that year, three months before my mom. Esther hadn't had the energy to write my mom while she was still alive. Bill was ten years younger than my mom and was one of her ministers. She truly loved both Bill and Esther and had no idea that Bill had passed when he unexpectedly appeared in the room.

I guessed that one by one the visitors were leaving, as she would call out, "I'll be with you soon, Mom and Dad. Thanks for coming everyone. It won't be long until I am with you."

They all must have left, for she then turned her head in the direction of where she had told me Dad was standing. "Honey, you stay here with me. I need you to be with me every single minute." She then closed her eyes and fell into a deep, soundless sleep.

I sat for a very long time in the silence of the room contemplating all that happened which I was aware of only through my mother's voice. I had never met my grandparents and yet they had been in the room with me. One of my favorite aunts, Aunt Almeda, had died ten years before. I had never gotten to say good-bye to her and missed her dearly. According to my mom, she was right next to me in the room wanting to talk to me. I felt privileged to have been a part of this special party.

My mom slept very peacefully for three hours. I sat right next to her. I didn't want to miss any more of her visitors. At 6:30 in the evening, she suddenly opened her eyes and seemed surprised to see me. The first words out of her mouth were, "Joyce, I love you so much. Thank you so much for letting me stay home to die. I'm so happy in my own home." Then she looked at me with a very deep, meaningful gaze. Her eyes were crystal clear and I felt like I was looking into the eyes of an enlightened saint. I have never seen her eyes so clear as she slowly and clearly spoke, "I am so happy with my dying process. It's just the way I wanted it to be."

Then she smiled her huge smile and said, "This is such a special day for me, and I feel so good. I want to have another party." I called over to Barry and he quickly came to be with us. I couldn't get Rami or Mira on the phone, so I called our friend Judy DeSimone. Judy visited my mom every week, bringing her cookies, books to read and in general bringing joy and happiness. She was like a cheerleader for my mom, always encouraging her. The three of us huddled around my mom's hospital bed for one and a half hours while she shared her wisdom with us. "This world has much to offer, but giving and receiving love is the most important. When you get close to the end of your life like me, you'll be grateful for all the love that you gave and received. Nothing is more important."

Judy was quite concerned about her cat's lack of appetite, and shared this with my mother. My mother's response was, "Judy, focus on the most important thing in life. You are loved! I have seen today that God is taking care of us all of the time. You don't have to worry."

Judy then asked, "Louise, can you tell us about where you're going?"

My mother answered, "The home we are going to is so beautiful, so special, so filled with love. There is more love than we can even possibly imagine here on earth."

The three of us felt bathed in her love. We laughed a lot and it felt as if my mother was a much younger woman now filled with an infinite wisdom. Her eyes stayed radiantly bright, as did her smile. I felt filled with joy as I gazed into her penetrating blue eyes.

The only other times in my life that I had felt this completely filled with love were the home births of our three children. Birth and death, the entry into and exit out of life, were bringing the same feeling of expansion of the heart. Looking into my mother's eyes felt exactly the same to me as looking into each newborn baby of mine.

Suddenly my mother smiled a big smile and said, "Aren't parties fun when there's a lot of love?"

Barry's note: It is quite common for a dying person to suddenly seem to come to life with renewed energy and mental clarity, days or weeks before their passing. Some explain it as a spiritual influx, or an opening of the connection between this life and the next. Regardless of why it happens, it does happen, and can last anywhere from a few minutes to many hours. Family and loved ones can even be fooled into the false hope of a miraculous healing. Anyone who works with the dying has seen this phenomenon and is amazed every time it happens.

For Louise, this was one of these times. Joyce and I could hardly believe it at first. One moment she looked like she was dying, barely able to move in her hospital bed. And then suddenly there she was, not only in her relatively awake condition from recent weeks, even months, but fully animated. It was as if she suddenly became younger by about five years. The physical transformation, with her lively head and hand movements, was incredible to watch. I fully expected her to leap out of bed and start dancing.

I sat close to her and took her hands in mine. She looked deeply and lovingly into my eyes with a gaze steadied by full consciousness. She told me how much she loved me, and how important I had been in her life. I nearly felt overwhelmed by the depth of love she was directing my way.

Somehow, although it was just Joyce, Judy and me, it felt like a grand party, a celebration of love. The little living room felt crowded with those who were celebrating Louise's earth life and impending transition to another life.

Judy said her farewell and left, and gradually Louise seemed to slip back into a body and mind that were not long for this world. Although there were other times of "spiritual influx," this particular time touched my heart the most deeply. I had a brief, but memorable, glimpse at what might be in store for a ninety-year-old, well-loved and respected woman no longer weighed down by a limited body and mind. But more important was a glimpse into my own life and death, the power of love, the joy of service, and my own soul's journey on this earth.

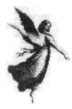

My mother closed her eyes after about an hour, and Judy and Barry left. I sat next to her, recording this wonderful event. A few minutes later, when it was just the two of us, she opened her eyes and softly said, "My mother always helped me in my life, and I will always help you in yours. Right now you have to take care of me, but soon I'll be able to take care of you. You'll know when I am there." We then held each other in a warm and loving embrace.

My mother and I sat for a while just looking into each other's eyes. I realized that I was not saying good-bye to *her*. I was just saying good-bye to a worn-out old body that didn't work anymore. My mother's love would always be with me.

While looking into her eyes, they suddenly darted across the room. "What is it, Mom?"

"Oh, it's just my angel again. She wants me to get ready." Her face suddenly became very determined as she slowly spoke, "Joyce there's one more thing I want you to promise me to do. This is very important to me."

I nodded to her and said, "Of course, Mother."

"Joyce, I want you to tell everyone you see that death is beautiful. Perhaps you could even write another book. Tell everyone not to be afraid. God loves us so much. This love is with us throughout our lives, but it is especially clear when a person dies. I never knew I could feel as much love as I have today, but also these past two weeks. You must do this for me!"

I hugged my mother tightly and said, "You are such a beautiful mother. I'll tell everyone what you've said. Who knows, maybe I will write a book about your dying process. I'll tell them all about this special party you had today."

My mother smiled her sun-like smile and, with a satisfied look, said, "Yes!" Then she closed her eyes and drifted off to sleep.

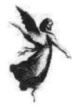

It is not unusual for a dying person to see loved ones that have passed on before. Two days before my dad suddenly died, he woke up and saw both of his deceased parents in his room with their arms outstretched in an act of welcoming him. He was only able to see them for a few minutes, but it made a big impression on him. As soon as my mother awoke in the morning, he excitedly told her about the visit and how happy it had made him. At that time my father was challenged with heart disease, but he was still working in his wood shop and was quite active. Even at age eighty-nine he was a dedicated engineer and relied on science and math. He would never make up something like that visit unless he had actually seen his parents.

One woman I know sat with her sister while she was dying. Right before she died, she sat up with a radiant glow on her face and said, "Sis, I can see Mom and Dad and Grandma and Grandpa. They are here to welcome me." Then she died.

Final Instructions – August 22

RAMI NOW DECIDED TO SLEEP IN THE SAME ROOM with Grandma every night until she passed. She told me that, right before I came over at 6:30AM, Grandma suddenly became very alert, looked up at the ceiling, smiled and said, "Thank you so much for telling me. So I don't have to hold my breath in. I just let it out all the way." Then with a very jubilant and triumphant voice she called out, "THANK YOU, THANK YOU, THANK YOU! Now I know what to do." Apparently, my mother had just received some very important instructions on dying.

I entered the room right after this happened and noticed a look of complete and utter contentment on my mother's face. She was unresponsive for the rest of that day. Carol, her wonderful hospice nurse, told me that she might die that night. She had received her final instructions on how to die, and now she was ready.

Singing in the Rain – August 23

RAMI HAD SLEPT IN THE ROOM WITH MY MOM. We all fully expected that she would pass that night. Rami told me she would call if she sensed something. I slept with the phone on my pillow. It never rang.

At six in the morning, I rose, quickly put on my clothes, and went over to my mom's apartment. I walked with a heavy step. Was my mother already dead? Was this the day she would die? I opened her apartment door slowly, not knowing what to expect. If someone had asked me what I was anticipating, I might have listed one hundred things, but never what I actually found.

When she saw me, she belted out, "Singing in the rain, I'm singing in the rain. What a glorious feeling, I'm happy again!" It was one of her favorite songs. Never mind that it hadn't rained for months.

Rami walked past me with tired, bloodshot eyes and moaned, "I'm going to try to get some sleep. Grandma has been singing all night. By the way, she pulled off her shirt."

I thanked Rami and walked closer to inspect my mom. She'd somehow thrown off her shirt and sheet and was lying without any clothes. For the past week

VISSELL

she had barely been able to pick up her arm. Yesterday she hadn't moved at all. How did she find the strength to actually pull off her shirt? In total confusion I asked her, "Mom why did you take off your beautiful shirt?"

She started to laugh and said, "Oh, you never know about me, the next thing you know you'll come and find a man in bed with me!" Then she looked up at the ceiling and said, "Don't worry, Hank, I'm just kidding Joyce." My mother always had a good sense of humor. Then she resumed "Singing in the Rain."

Susie arrived and I noticed from the slow and deliberate way she was walking over to the apartment that she, too, expected my mom to have died that night. She was in for a big surprise as well. When she tentatively entered the room, my mother again broke into, "Singing in the rain, I'm singing in the rain. What a glorious feeling, I'm happy again!"

Susie broke into a wide smile and quickly stepped into service mode. She gave my mother a bed bath and all the other wonderful things that made my mother clean and comfortable. My mom then slept for several hours and I sat in the room with her while she slept.

Around noon she woke with a start and started singing again. Then she said, "I must call Bruce and John-Nuri." This whole day was unprecedented, so I figured why not. I dialed my brother's cell phone and got him just as he was about to teach a class to his graduate electrical engineering students at the University of Minnesota. I knew my brother was expecting a call that Mom had died, so I softly told him, "Bruce, Mom wants to say one more thing to you." She serenaded him loudly with "Singing in the rain," ending with, "My dying process is all very exciting. I love you, Bruce."

After that she said, "That was fun, now dial up John-Nuri." I hesitated, but she insisted. Who am I to argue with a dying mother and grandmother? I got John-Nuri as he was putting the final touches on packing for the college river trip. We caught him just in time. He would have been off and out of cell phone range in just a few minutes. My mom took the phone from me and yet again launched into her loud song, ending with, "This is so exciting, John-Nuri! I love you."

I sometimes wonder what that experience was like for Bruce and John-Nuri, seeing on their cell phone that the call was from us, expecting the news that she had died, only to hear her loudly singing, "Singing in the rain. What a glorious feeling. I'm happy again."

I sat with my mother for several hours. Over and over again she had me sing her Louise song. I started to yawn. I wanted to be there for her, but I was getting tired.

Finally she said, "Joyce, I want a *real* visitor!" Part of me felt a little hurt that she didn't consider me a real visitor, but the greater part of me felt perplexed. How was I supposed to find a "real visitor" at such short notice? I happened to look out the window and saw Rami's friend, Chris Lepisto, washing his truck in our driveway. Chris was visiting for a few days from Colorado. He is a naturopathic doctor and a very fun person. My mother had never met him before.

I yelled out the window to him, "Chris, do you have time to visit with my mother for a little bit right now?" Without hesitating, he put down the hose and ran up the stairs. "Mom, this is Rami's friend, Chris." She greeted him like he was a long lost friend.

As I said before, my mother loved to make new friends. And here she was, shortly before her death, doing what she loved the most, making a new friend. Chris and my mom sat together for over an hour, singing old Broadway tunes together. Who could imagine such a scene as part of her dying process?

After Chris left, I checked on her again. She was beaming and said, "I feel so happy I got to make a new friend. We had a lot of fun." Her eyes then darted across the room.

"Mom, what is it?"

"It's my angel again. She says I really need to stop singing and get ready now."

Curious, I asked her, "Mom, what does your angel look like?"

She looked in the direction of where her angel was and said, "Well, she doesn't have any wings. She's just bright and shining, and there's so much love coming from her. I can't see her face."

"Mother, why don't you ask to see her face," I urged.

My mother looked back in the same direction as before, and I could see her lips moving. Tears formed in her eyes and then spilled down her cheeks as she responded:

"My angel's face is my mother's face. My mother is my angel taking care of me and bringing me back home."

She then closed her eyes with a look of happiness upon her face.

I sat for a long time pondering my mother's "angel," *my grandmother.* How wonderful for my mother to feel so cared for and protected in this precious time of her death.

A Church Made of People – August 24

AFTER YESTERDAY MORNING, I seriously didn't know what to expect when I walked into my mother's apartment. As I woke at 6AM, quickly dressing to relieve Rami, I wondered what I would find. Yesterday I expected that she might have died, only to find that she had thrown off her shirt and was singing at the top of her lungs. I tried to prepare myself for the unexpected.

Rami looked exhausted as she gathered her things and quickly left, saying, "I hardly slept at all. Grandma was talking all night about wanting to go to church."

As Rami closed the door behind her, I walked over to my mom.

"Did you keep Rami up all last night?" I asked.

Her sweet, childlike, innocent face looked up at me as she said, "Oh, no, I slept the entire night."

I was struck by how completely lovable she appeared. As she was looking into my eyes, her eyes suddenly darted to the left. "Joyce, my beautiful mother angel is here again. She is telling me that I must hurry. I don't have much more time." Then a look of worry crossed her face as she said, "You must take me to my church right away. How can I take the hand of God without being in my church? Hurry, please, I must go to church right now."

"Mom, I can't take you to church. It's impossible," I tried to explain. It would have taken an ambulance to get her to church, and the movement would have caused unbearable pain for her.

"Joyce, you must honor this final request. I must go to church right now."

How can I argue with my dying mother? What am I to do? Suddenly an idea crosses my mind and I say to her, "All right Mom, I'll take you right now, but first I need you to just sit up."

"Well, that's easy for me. I'll do it right now," she said with confidence. I watched as nothing happened. After a few minutes she announced, "Well, I guess I can't do that anymore. You're right, I can't go to church right now." She lay back in bed, a troubled look on her face.

Susie came in then and did all the extra things she does to make my mother feel clean and cared for. After she left, my mother slept for five hours.

I was over at my home for a short while when I heard a knock on the door. Emily, my mother's Hospice chaplain, was there to tell me that my mother was awake now and seemed very agitated. "She wants to go to church," Emily reported.

"Oh no, not that again," I thought as I went over with her.

As soon as my mom saw me enter her apartment, she called out with a sense of urgency, "Joyce, you must take me to my church. I don't have much time. I have to go. Do anything you can to get me there."

Emily stepped forward and asked, "Louise, why is church so important right now?

"Church is my other family. I need my spiritual family right now."

Then I got it, church for her wasn't about the building; church was about the people. I left Emily with my mom and ran home to find her church's directory. I quickly made several calls and got two wonderful couples from the church to agree to come within a half hour, Marion and Jess, and David and Joyce, all in their seventies. Unfortunately, Bob Bowles was out of town on that day, so he couldn't come.

Within half an hour my mother had her church. These wonderful four people, along with Barry and me, had church for my mother. We sang her favorite hymns, spoke the 23rd Psalm, and ended with the Lord's Prayer. My mother was radiant the whole time. She was in her church. Her final request was met. She was extremely happy.

When we finished, she smiled at all of us and said, "Thank you, and I love you so much. Now I can take the hand of God. Thank you for helping make my journey so peaceful and loving. And thank you for bringing my church right here."

After her "church" left, my mother and I sat for a while just looking into each other's eyes. Finally, she spoke to me one last time.

"My mother never left me after she died and I will never leave you, Joyce. Whenever you need to feel me, you will hear me speak to you within your heart. I have loved my dying process. I'm ready to go now and feel very happy."

She then closed her eyes for the last time.

For the next two hours, with eyes closed, she softly spoke the following words with long pauses in between:

"It's so beautiful!
Thank you for coming for me.
I never dreamed it would be so wonderful.
There is so much light.
Hank, Mom, Dad, I'm coming.
I feel so loved. There's more love than I ever imagined.
I'm coming! I'm coming! I'm so happy."

I sat with my mother for the rest of the evening. A look of complete fulfillment was upon her face. During the pauses between speaking, she would lift one of her arms and reach her hand toward something as if to hold on. It was quite clear to me that she was fulfilling what she said she would do in her last words to us, take the loving hand of her Creator. I knew that my mother would soon make her triumphant march to heaven.

Eventually my mother became very still. I believe that some essential part of her had really left her body at this point. From then on, moving her body caused no reaction in her face. It was now time for her body to completely wind down and allow her to fully go. Her breathing came slower and slower. I had been sitting with her since 6:30 that morning, and it was now 10:30 at night. Part of me wanted to stay at her bedside until the very end, but I was fatigued in a way I rarely get. It felt as if every part of my being was completely spent. It's a good thing to realize your limitations in a situation like this.

I called Rami and she agreed to spend yet another night with Grandma. I hardly even remember my head touching down on my pillow that night.

The Day of Puffs – August 25

RAMI STAYED WITH GRANDMA ALL NIGHT, with strict instructions to call me if it looked like Grandma was taking her last breath. The phone never rang. I was awake before the sun rose, quickly dressed and walked over to Mom's apartment. What would this day be like?

It did not surprise me to find that Rami was exhausted from the night. As she gathered her things she explained to me, "Grandma looks like she is about to die any minute, but she doesn't. I'm beyond tired. I've got to get a little sleep. Call me if anything happens." Then she trudged out the door.

I went over and sat with my mother. She was totally unresponsive. Her breaths were coming every minute or every minute and a half. When Susie walked in to bathe my mother she took one look and said, "I won't be caring for her today. Your mother is going to die very shortly. She is a good woman, and I have totally enjoyed being able to care for her."

With tears in our eyes, Susie and I hugged goodbye. Susie gave my mother such love and attention, and was a bright spot in the morning for both of us. I will always be grateful to her for all that she did.

Barry and Mira joined me shortly after Susie left. We sat on the couch next to her hospital bed, ready for her to take her last breath. Bob Bowles, my mom's minister, came to say prayers for her. As he left, he told us it probably would be a very short time now. I called my brother and told him. A weekend Hospice nurse came to check on her and told me she was amazed that my mother didn't die last night, as her vital signs were barely present. As she left, she said it might be within the hour. She asked if we wanted her to stay, but I told her we preferred to be alone with my mom.

The hour passed, and then another, and yet another. Her breaths had longer and longer intervals between them. Just when we thought she had taken her last breath, another would come in a short "puff." Barry, Mira and I told my mom how much we loved her, and that it was okay for her to go to her new home.

The same breathing pattern continued all day. Finally, Mira wandered over to our home and her old room for a break. Barry needed a break, too, and returned to our home, promising to bring over my dinner.

I stayed and watched her breathing pattern. Why was it going this way? I was reminded of my labor experience with our first child, Rami. I had prepared and planned and knew exactly the way I wanted it to be.

But it didn't go that way at all. With birth and death, there needs to be enormous surrender to how the process will unfold. I always pictured my mother looking at us as she took her last breath, but that was not to be. She basically was gone, but her body was still "puffing" breath in its own strange pattern.

Around 7PM, I was burned out. I had been with my mom for over thirteen hours, just watching her breathing. After each short puff I thought it might be the end, only to see another puff one and a half minutes later.

Finally, I called Hospice and said I needed help. In a very short time, another weekend nurse showed up at my mom's apartment. This woman's name was Dawn. She was our age, had long, graying hair and was obviously of hippy vintage. I felt a connection with her right away. Barry and Mira joined us shortly after. The four of us sat around my mom's hospital bed and talked about death. It was one of those evenings I will never forget. It felt as if we were in a timeless, spacious place far away from the realities of the world, where the only thing that mattered was birth, love, and death. The sound of my mother's puffs added a touching poignancy to this other-worldly conversation.

At one point in that evening, Emily called to find out how my mother was doing. She wondered if my mother was not dying because she needed to say good-bye to my brother Bruce. I called my brother in Minnesota and told him I would be putting the phone to mom's ear and that he should say good-bye. I held the phone to her ear and listened myself while he said the most beautiful things to her, encouraging her to let go and reach for God. Surely, I thought, she would go now. But her breathing pattern continued.

I went outside and found my mother's cat, Ben. Ben had not been allowed to be with my mother, because one tiny scratch from him could cause her to bleed for days. Her skin was that frail. This night, however, Ben was allowed full access to the apartment. He stretched out next to her chest and purred the loudest I have ever heard him.

"Puff," and a minute and a half later, "puff." Purr, purr, purr and puff, these sounds filled the air. Dawn was a total angel when we desperately needed one. She gave us permission to relax, and not be so anxious about being there when my mother actually took her last breath. Barry, Mira, Rami and I were all wiped out. Not one of us had the strength to keep watch with my mom anymore. Dawn suggested that we all go to sleep and let Ben continue the watch. She hugged us good-bye and left. Mira and Barry left as well. I spoke some final words to my mom and reluctantly left the room. I felt completely exhausted.

Ben looked proud to be able to be with my mother. He had been my mom's very best friend before her weakening skin would not allow him to be close. He was my dad's cat originally and then was adopted by my mom when my dad died. Ben and my mom had quite a loving, close relationship. He seemed to understand the importance of this night, and that he had been entrusted with a very important job. He would keep vigil with constant purrs.

The Hallelujah Chorus – August 26

IT WAS SO HARD TO LEAVE MY MOTHER that last night. I had such a strong desire to be right there when she took her final breath. But I was beyond tired. I slept a little, then woke and started walking over to her apartment. As I was climbing the stairs I heard a loud motor going. "Oh, no," I thought, "we must have left a motor running by mistake." I opened the door to her apartment, and there in the glow of the soft night light I spotted Ben. The motor I heard was his loud purring. He was taking his job very seriously and was giving my mother all he could. He lay on top of her, protecting his precious owner.

My mother was still in her same breathing pattern, one breath every one and a half minutes. She was completely unresponsive and her ankles were growing purple from lack of oxygen. I kissed her, and sat with her for a while, but the complete, deep fatigue I felt would not allow me to stay in the room. Ben looked at me as if to say, "Go and sleep. I have everything covered here."

I left and walked back down the stairs, hearing the loud purring as I walked. I have never heard Ben purr so loudly, before or since.

I awoke very early the next day, and Barry and I both went over to see my mother. Surely she must have died in the middle of the night. Climbing the stairs, I heard the familiar puff. We entered the room. It had now been thirty hours. I had been so strong for my mother this whole year, and yet now in the very hours before her death I totally fell apart. I cried and Barry held me. I just didn't think I had it in me to sit another whole day listening to that breathing pattern. I wanted so much to be there for my mother, but I just couldn't. I felt like a well that had run dry—at the most important time. Barry told me to do something special for myself, and he would sit with my mother until I came home.

I went swimming. It was the strangest thing. I hadn't driven away from our home in over a week in my total focus on being with my mother. Here she was, possibly taking her last breath, and I was driving away. It felt unreal, and yet I knew I had to get away. Swimming has always been a very spiritual thing for me. There is something about being in the water that helps me to feel close to God. Swimming in a lake, when there is light on the water from a sunrise, is probably my favorite thing to do. Today I was just swimming in a pool, fifteen minutes away from our house. Fortunately, it was early in the day and no one else was there. As I was swimming, I heard my mother's voice telling me to have a good time. She said she was waiting for me. I had a premonition that she would die at 1PM.

I drove home, took a shower, put on special clothes and went over to relieve Barry. I felt strong and centered, better than I had felt in several days. Barry left and I sat with my mother. Her breath now came every two minutes. I felt her death was imminent. In my heart I could clearly hear her talking with me:

"Joyce, please remember our love is forever.

I didn't want to die until you felt strong and rested and could hear me speaking to you.

My new home is amazing and more beautiful than you can ever imagine."

Please tell everyone you know that death can be so beautiful. This is the most important thing to me.

After this was "said," her breaths became even shallower. She had told me to put on the Hallelujah Chorus from Handel's Messiah while she breathed her final breaths. She wanted to triumphantly march to her new home. I went and put on the music very loudly. Even though she had been unresponsive for over thirty-six hours, her mouth clearly shaped into a smile.

Then she took her last breath. I held her and told her how happy I was for her.

Barry heard the music and came running over. We sat quietly with her while the music played. I felt her taking the hand of God while she joyfully marched. When the music ended, I read again her favorite story about dying from Henry Van Dyke:

I am standing upon the seashore. A ship spreads her white sails to the morning breeze and starts for the blue ocean. She is an object of beauty and strength. I stand and watch her until at length she hangs like a speck of white cloud just where the sea and sky come to mingle with each other.

Then someone at my side says: "There she is gone!"

"Gone where?"

Gone from my sight. That is all. She is just as large in mast and hull and spar as she was when she left my side and she is just as able to bear her load of living freight to her destined port.

Her diminished size is in me, not in her. And just at the moment when someone at my side says, "There she is gone!" there are other eyes watching her coming, and other voices ready to take up the glad shout: "Here she comes!"

And that is dying.

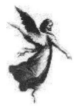

I called my brother right away. He hadn't slept a wink all night and was so relieved when I called. He promised to call all of our many relatives. After that, Barry and I sat a long time with my mother, talking to her gently and telling her how happy we were for her. I could just imagine her complete joy. Then Barry started to sing to her.

While he was singing, tears flowed down my cheeks. Barry reached over and held me. I allowed myself to be held like a little child whose mommy had just died. I had been strong for these many long months, supporting my mother in all of her changes and in the final two weeks being excited for her as she requested. It felt so healing to just let the tears flow and allow the little child in me to have expression. For though my mother's death was beautiful in every way, I would still miss her dearly. I felt extremely happy for her and transformed by all that I had been privileged to witness during her dying process. But I am also a human being, and will grieve her absence from my life. As Barry was holding me, I felt my mother's arms around me, reminding me of her promise to never leave me. I could hear her words in my heart:

"My dear daughter, now I get to take care of you again. I will be right there waiting when you make your triumphant march back home. Thank you for all you did to allow me to have such a beautiful death."

The room felt charged with love, and I felt a deep peace sweep over me.

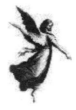

I called Hospice to tell them that my mother had died and that I wanted a nurse to come to the house. Within an hour, a different weekend nurse appeared at our doorstep. Each and every Hospice person that came to our home was absolutely lovely and compassionate in every way. This nurse was no exception. Most of the other Hospice people wore simple professional clothes, but this nurse had her own style. She showed up in a beautiful dress and high heels, looking like she was going out on the town rather than tending to a departed old woman. She was very compassionate and understanding that my mom had just passed. But she was also upbeat in a way that was delightful.

She announced in a no-nonsense way, "Let's get your mom looking beautiful!"

Barry excused himself, and the two of us headed up to where my mother's body lay. The nurse gently ordered me about to find my mother's favorite clothes. Then she went looking in the bathroom closet for powder and added, "All women your mother's age love powder. Let's get her smelling good." She found some powder I didn't even know Mom had and got to work. She totally cleaned my mother, and powdered her body. Then she dressed her in the clothes I had picked out, her Sunday best. She fussed over her hair as if she were a hairdresser. Then she applied lipstick and just a bit of rouge and my mother looked like she was ready for a special event at church.

When she was done with my mother, this beautifully-dressed nurse stepped back, took a long look, and said, "I've worked for Hospice a long time now. I've taken care of a lot of patients when they die. The expressions on a person's face after they die tell me how they have lived their life. Some people die with worry lines, and some with expressions of fear or pain. Your mother has a look of complete fulfillment. I can tell she lived her life well." She showed me what she was looking at, and I could see the most serene expression of contentment on my mother's face.

My mother did live her life in fulfillment. Her mission in this life was really quite simple: to be a friend to all people and to give her love. She was the friendliest, most loving person that I have ever met. The loving kindness she showed others was its own reward. The body she left behind as she marched back home reflected a woman who had finished her mission and was at peace with its completion.

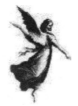

Later, while I was out walking our dogs with Barry, Rami and her friends, Josie and Amy, arrived with armloads of flowers. They proceeded up to my mother's apartment and placed the flowers all around her body and in the room. It looked like she was lying in a fairy garden.

That evening, Barry and I, Rami and Mira sat in her apartment for a long time talking about my mother. She looked so beautiful with flowers all around her in the light of many candles. There seemed to be magic in the air as we all so strongly felt Grandma's presence. She was loving and thanking each one of us for our care and love of her. The four of us felt a deep peace in our hearts. We had each sacrificed a lot of time and energy to be able to lovingly care for her over the past year. Through that giving, we had helped her to pass from this world in such a special way. In this time of her death, we each felt very satisfied that we had served her fully. We harbored no regrets. We each knew we had done all we could, and that feeling brought such peace over the months following her death.

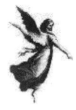

Two days after my mother died, I was sitting with Barry high up on the bleachers of the sports arena at

Lewis and Clark College where our son was beginning his freshman year. Not knowing if we would be able to leave my mother, we had made flight reservations anyway many months ago to attend the opening ceremony for freshman students.

We chose to sit away from the other families as I was still feeling quite vulnerable. It was a shock to go from my mother's death bed to this maze of excited freshman. Part of me just wanted to be alone at home, or just sitting quietly in my mom's apartment. But I also wanted to be here for John-Nuri. I seemed caught between two worlds.

Parent orientation was high energy with lots of people, a stark contrast to the last few days spent with my mom. Now the final ceremony was to begin. First, the college faculty walked out dressed in their robes. It was very impressive. Then, to the tune of a triumphant march, the new college freshman walked out in a long line. John-Nuri had come from a graduating class of fourteen students. Now he was one of five hundred. Barry and I strained to see him. "Yes," I heard myself excitedly call out, "There he is, the tallest one!" We started to cheer loudly. At this very moment, I felt a distinct presence right next to me, cheering him on as well. It was so strong that I looked to my left to see who it was. There was only an empty space. I realized it was my mother. I hadn't felt her presence since the day she died, and yet here she was cheering on the grandson she loved so much, just as she had promised to do.

Intimate With Death – Rami Vissell

PERHAPS YOU HAVE A GRANDMA? Maybe you had a grandma? Maybe you had a pet, a parent, or a loved one that has passed on? I wonder if you have met death. I met death. It was not the terrible and tragic experience I have sometimes imagined death to be. It was at times a spiritual journey, a bundle of laughs, an otherworldly adventure, a cherished gift, and a deep look into myself and my own mortality.

I want to tell you the story of my grandma and me. My grandma was very involved in my life right from the beginning. She cared for me and my sister when my parents were away working for two weeks each summer. She fed me delicious food, and even better desserts. She sang to me, took me to a place called "Art Park," and let me eat ice cream in a real cone. As I grew older, she was always there for important events and fascinated me with stories of her life back when she was a little girl.

Fifteen years ago, my grandparents moved into a garage apartment right next to my parent's house. When I started college twelve years ago, I moved into a little cabin not far from my parents' property. So I have always had the luxury to walk a few minutes through

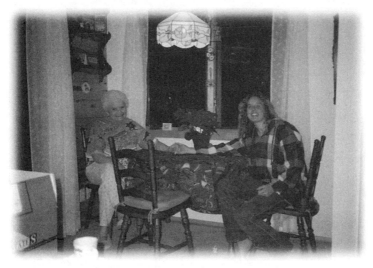

Louise and Rami holding hands in her apartment in 1994.

the woods and up a hill to Grandma's house. I have never taken for granted this closeness to my grandma. I felt so lucky. I could stop by any time for tea and cookies… and I did often, because they were so yummy. Grandma would do most of the talking, and I would listen eagerly. I loved hearing how her family would heat up bricks on the coal stove, then put them in a sock and tuck them in each child's bed for warmth on cold nights.

Eight years ago, my grandpa passed on. I was very close to him as well. We loved to build things out of wood in his workshop. Mostly, as grandpa put it, "We made a lot of sawdust, and made small ones out of big ones," and laughed a lot. I remember the sad day my sister and I were at my parent's house when my grandma breathlessly exclaimed over the phone that grandpa had fallen and was dead. We rushed next door to find grandpa unconscious on the floor. My sister and I did CPR on him until the ambulance arrived. The paramedics were impressed that we had maintained color in his skin by breathing for him but there was nothing more that could be done. It was a sudden and unexpected run-in with death.

I'd had some dear pets die, some childhood acquaintances, and my other grandpa a few years back. But this death hit me hard. One moment I was taking my grandpa to the lumber yard to listen to him talk shop with the guys and buy hardware for a project we were working on, the next ... he was dead. I was angry, devastated, sad, confused – the whole gamut of emotions that comes with great loss. Yes, he lived a good long life, but I was not ready to let him go. I never got to say good-bye. I had no regrets for I had loved him every moment we were together. But he was ripped from me and my family so quickly. In time I recovered, integrated him into my being, and had amazing dreams where he would come to me and tell me about the finer points of working with wood, how to use tools and, most importantly, that he loved me.

This was my experience of death – that it is quite sudden and leaves you very devastated and bewildered. I guess it was safe to say that I, like most people, did not like death and was afraid of it. Sure, I was comforted as a child with images of angels, a heavenly presence that is always there, and a peaceful place where we go to be free of suffering and despair. But this did not resolve the mystery and unease I felt about death. I just didn't really know it, this process called death. This dramatically changed for me with the death of my grandma.

A little over a year ago, my grandma started her "decline," as some would say. She gradually was unable to care for her basic needs. She could not move about her apartment, go to the bathroom nor feed herself. She was losing her independence, and eventually became totally dependent on our family for care. This was a real hard blow for her. She kept saying she did not want to burden anyone.

At that time I was working two jobs. I had established my private practice as a therapist working with teens and families, and I was also working for a mental health agency. Our family had a serious meeting about Grandma. We talked about how friends and family had recommended placing her in a nursing home. My grandma could go into one of these places and have all her needs met, and we as a family could go about our life as normal, not being burdened with the responsibility of caring for her. It just didn't feel right. We wanted Grandma to stay at home. I cut down my hours at the agency. My sister and parents adjusted their schedules as well.

Once we put some effort into a plan, it worked. We were all on a schedule. We had good communication about Grandma's needs and came up with creative solutions to every challenge that arose. I took my new responsibility seriously. It was not difficult waking up my sweet grandma in the morning. She always greeted me with a huge smile. I would walk into her room singing and she would join me with her frail sweet voice. Like any other person needing to complain from time to time about this or that, my grandma would sometimes protest having to take a shower, or taking the many pills in her cupboard. But most of the time she was quite pleasant and grateful to receive our care.

If it was shower day, I would bathe her and marvel at her body. Her body was so beautiful to me. It had carried her for ninety years through life. And like any ninety-year-old piece of fine machinery, her body was starting to shut down.

Each Wrinkle Tells a Story
— Rami Vissell

You have returned to me like a child.
Where once you held me as a baby,
now I am the careful hands that hold you.
Your eyes are the same,
glinting with mystery, love, and deep knowing.
You have walked for 90 years upon the earth.
Innocence has become wisdom.
Questions have become answers.
Smooth complexion has become a rough landscape of can-
yons and mountains.
Beauty has become something deeper.
You let me wash your body on Wednesdays and Saturdays
if the heat is turned up high, and you can have a cookie befo-
rehand.
Do you really know how beautiful you are?
Each wrinkle tells a story.
How much you laughed, how you loved,
where you rested, how you dressed, how little you frowned.
Your skin is like a fine silk dress,
worn and washed so often because it was so loved.
Now it is fragile to the touch, and soft, and familiar
and just as beautiful as the day you put it on.

Most sunny warm mornings I would bundle her up like there was a blizzard outside and take her to the beach. I would push her in her wheelchair for about a quarter of a mile each way on the path by the beach. She would not let a single person pass by without saying "Hi" and "How are you?" She smiled her biggest smile no matter who happened to be passing her by. Of course the regulars knew her by name and loved her as if she were their own grandmother. I marveled at and learned from her compassion.

A few months after I had started caring for my grandma, my fiancé, River, left me. Like my previous experience of death, this experience was sudden, unexpected, and devastating. I was so sad and cried all the time. My grandma, in her infinite wisdom and sweetness, listened to me and loved me and then said, "Now it's just you and me, kid. We can pretend we're an old married couple." We both laughed very hard, but there was real truth in that for me. I needed her companionship more than ever and she gave it without question. I wasn't the only one doing the caring. It was very mutual.

I felt really devastated about this breakup because, at age thirty-one, I had been feeling the intense desire to be a mother, and getting married was a big step in that direction for me. When my fiancé left, my dreams of being a mom anytime soon seemed shattered. Again, my grandma, in her infinite wisdom, without even knowing I had really wanted to be a mom, said, "You're getting practice caring for me, so one day when you have kids, you will make the best mom!" And that was the healing for me. My pain was great with the loss of my love, but having my grandma to care for filled a deep void for me. We needed each other and committed ourselves to the healing of the other in a perfect way.

The hardest part about caring for my grandma in the beginning had nothing to do with her or the caring. It was the constant bombardment from friends about why our family was not putting her in a home. Some of my friends asked why I was "wasting" my precious time caring for my grandma when someone else could do all the "dirty" work and I could just visit her. My peers and colleagues questioned me giving up some of my agency hours to care for my grandma. They would downright tease me that while they were going on to get their licenses and high-paying jobs, I was "wiping my grandma's butt and missing out on life." I was missing out on life? Or were they missing out on life? It really got me thinking about our culture and what we do with death.

Many of us don't want death around. We push it away, far away. We advertise and promote youth, and we shun any qualities that point to old age. Wrinkles are bad, sagging is bad, graying is bad. Don't get me started! But putting our elderly in homes and forgetting about them? That's so sad. Like I said, I had a very strong idea about death, and I didn't like it. But all that changed when my grandma passed on and gave me the greatest gift ever – her final gift.

The ease of caring for my grandma eventually gave way to the final weeks before her passing, which were more difficult. Grandma, who never really complained at all, started experiencing some major pain in her body. It was hard to see my beloved grandma become so fragile and in pain right before my eyes. Fortunately, Hospice Caring Project came in and helped a lot. We as a family got a whole education on bed sores, medications, treatments, exercises, how to lift a body that could not lift itself and so on.

The last few weeks, I spent a lot of time with Grandma. She could not get out of her apartment and really did not want to get out of bed. I read to her, sang to her, talked to her. She had become much more introspective and focused more on things she felt were important. For example, she could never accept River's and my breakup. No matter how I answered that question she would always say, "I like River a lot. I believe you both should be together."

The beauty of this ever more difficult situation was that my family and I were constantly adapting our strategies and applying our ideas for things to run smoother. As each new challenge with Grandma's failing body arose, we were there to meet it as a team. It was sometimes difficult. We all had our moments of sadness at the inevitable end.

What would happen in the end? How would she die? Would I come to wake her in the morning and find she had died in her sleep? I would talk to her about death and this whole process. My mom told me one day that Grandma had told her, "I'm happy with my dying process."

Indeed, my grandma's dying process was a gift to all of us in the family. In the last week before she passed on, she slowed considerably. She did not get out of bed, did not eat, did not talk much accept to unseen beings, and was transitioning out of this world and into the next. I slept every night right by her bed on the couch. I didn't exactly get the best sleep but the experience was otherworldly. All night I lay and listened to her carry on whole conversations with unseen and unheard (to me) beings. Sometimes I could tell she was speaking to my grandpa. It sounded like she was on the phone with him. She would tell him about how wonderful I was to take such good care of her, then pause for moments to listen to what he said and then respond laughing at a joke I was not privy to. It was just like my grandpa to make her laugh. The conversations were logical and precise. She was not babbling in a crazy delusional manner, but carrying on meaningful conversations. I just listened and felt privileged to be a witness.

Each night was an otherworldly adventure. I would strain to try to feel the beings that were obviously present in the room. Though I could not feel them, I did feel and sense my grandma's relief and comfort in her final days. She was surrounded by her family and friends both alive and not. It truly seemed like a massive graduation party was taking place. All were present to support and wish her well. I felt comforted, too. I could imagine that, in my own final hour, I would be surrounded by similar love for my ultimate step into the unknown. I believe now there is no such thing as being alone.

A few days before her body took its last breath, she looked at me with such love and said, "You don't need to worry about me. I'm going to be great. I'm looking forward to where I'm going next. I have no regrets, and I'll never forget you. A part of me will stay with you always." She communicated so clearly that she was not afraid and we should not grieve for her, but instead rejoice. After all, it was a graduation, a celebration of her life, a transition into the next phase.

I was at a friend's house in the afternoon on August 26, 2007, when my mom called and told me my grandma had taken her last breath and passed in the most peaceful way. I took this news outside and lay down by myself in the grass of an apple orchard. I spread my limbs out and felt the ground holding me. I looked up at the blue sky and felt heaven open up, that mysterious place of peace beyond our waking reality. I felt the spirit of my grandma, as expansive as the universe, reach down to touch me. It felt like a doorway opened in that moment and I could almost hear her say, "I will never leave you, my child. I am right here."

It was such a profound moment. It was timeless and utterly beautiful. Everything was so beautiful. I saw the apple trees, the grass, the sun, the birds, so clearly. I was in the moment and my grandma was there with me enjoying her new freedom.

I believe that death is not the end, but a transformation. We are like energy that is neither created nor destroyed, but just transformed into new form. I looked around now and I saw the beauty of my grandma everywhere. I felt her hold me through the soft grasses around me.

But my moment of connection to the universe and my grandma's expansive being came to an end. My thoughts took control: I need to cry. This is a sad time. I shouldn't feel so much joy.

The door closed. I was confused by these feelings. Shouldn't I be in pain, sobbing at my great loss? I felt guilty because I wanted to run through the field and yell to the world that I loved my grandma and I was so happy for her new-found freedom. She had graduated, earned her degree! I did feel the sadness of losing my companion for walks, talks, movies and singing in the rain, but I also was so at peace with it all. It was her time, and I had said my good-bye. I decided to run through the field, and as I did I felt great exhilaration for I knew my grandma was running right by my side.

The weeks and months that followed were a transition. I felt I was grieving, but I was also moving into accepting the change. My life had to change from waking Grandma up every morning, putting her to bed, feeding her, fussing over her, washing her clothes, counting her pills, laughing with her. I did cry at times, but it was more for the loss of this way of life I had come to cherish with her. My grief for my grandma was changing into joy. My friends couldn't understand why I didn't mope about. My family shared my same experience. We would get together and talk about the wonderful times we had with Grandma. We would remind each other of the funny moments with her and then we would all laugh.

Grandma taught me that death is not something to be feared, but embraced. It is not an end, but a trans-formation. And no matter what, we will not be alone, but will be surrounded by loved ones and love beyond imagination. I have no doubt my grandpa had the same experience of connection and love, but his was a lot more sudden. My grandma's dying experience was slowed down so my family and I could witness the process and understand the vast beauty that takes place in this final ceremony in body form.

PhD in Love

WE HAD MY MOTHER'S MEMORIAL SERVICE thirteen days after she died. This extra time allowed my brother and his oldest son to make travel arrangements.

A memorial service (or funeral ceremony) is a beautiful way to say good-bye and honor a departed loved one. I have known several people who have not wanted a memorial service. They figure they will be dead and don't want people standing around talking about them. In these families where there is no ceremony after a person dies, there is often a sense of emptiness, that something is incomplete. I have known people in such instances to have a memorial service years later, just to have that feeling of completeness.

My mother had planned her memorial service ten years before she died. Sally, the secretary at her church, had it on file. There in my mother's neat writing was all that she wanted. At the end of her writing was a little personal note to whomever would be reading it, "Remember, I want you to be happy for me!"

My mother's love had touched so many people in the fifteen years she lived in California that her little church was full. I noticed Pat was there with several of the "Wall Sitters" from her walks at Rio Del Mar Beach.

She had touched such a variety of people, and they all came to give their respects to a great lady. Everyone had a safe place within her heart.

Most people do not speak at a family member's memorial service, for they are afraid that they will just get up there and cry. I had all of those fears, but was determined to speak. I felt that speaking at her memorial service was an important gift I wanted to give to my mother. Though a shy person by nature, I have had to get used to speaking in public for our work. I usually prepare a speech just in my mind and then give it without notes. It is not such a big deal to me anymore. But to speak at my mother's memorial service was a very big deal. As a matter of fact, it was the biggest, scariest thing I could have done. I was afraid I would just crumble as soon as I walked up there. And then what would I do? Just stand up there in front of all those people and cry and stumble through a speech. Many people advised me not to do it.

I wrote out my talk which is something I never do. Then I went over and over and over it again and again. I knew it backwards and forwards. I practiced it in front of the dogs and then in front of the cats, who promptly fell asleep. I spoke loudly to the trees on our property, and then to my flowers. I said it before I went to sleep, and when I woke up. I figured that knowing it so well would be my safety.

When the time came to speak at the memorial service, I slowly walked up to the podium. I held onto that wooden box for all it was worth and I gave my talk, which was five minutes long. As I was speaking, I felt my mother's arms wrap around me and at the same time felt a strong energy of love come through me. People who have known me for a long time, and have heard me speak at other occasions, said it was by far the most beautiful talk I had ever given. Some shared that they could see a bright light around me as I was speaking, and some of these people were my mother's older friends who don't normally see or talk about such things. I was so grateful I had pushed past the huge fear within me and had given my love in words at her service.

Memorial Talk

I'VE ALWAYS BEEN VERY PROUD AND GRATEFUL to be able to call Louise my mother. In the few stories that I'll share, I hope you will feel my great love and respect for this remarkable woman.

Just between my father, brother, me, our spouses, and the grandchildren, there are three PhD's, one MD, several Masters' degrees, and all the rest have a college education, except for our son who has just started. My mother is the only one of us who just has a high school education. And yet with all these degrees in the family, my mother was without a doubt the wisest one, the one we would all turn to for direction and guidance. For my mother majored in the one subject that doesn't give a degree – love. She devoted her entire life to loving others.

While I was growing up in Buffalo, New York, my mother had many friends. All of these friends collected things: tea cups, bells, orchids, antiques, hats, and her best friend collected wigs. My mother told me she never wanted to collect things; she only wanted to collect friends. For my mom, life was filled with opportunities to make new friends. It didn't matter if the person had high prestige or was homeless. She treated all people with kindness and respect.

My mother lived in the apartment next to our home for fifteen years. Part of our work is counseling others. We have a steady stream of people coming to our home office. From her apartment window, my mom would sit and watch all of this, and one day opened the sliding door to her porch and invited a young man who had just finished his appointment to come up and have cookies and tea. The man grew to love his time with my mom so much that he came up after each session with Barry.

One day he told Barry that he felt he had gotten what he needed from the sessions. Then rather shyly he asked, "Is it all right if I continue to come and visit with your mother-in-law?" We always kidded her that she was going to put us out of business. That man was one of many who benefited from "cookies and love therapy."

Thirty years ago, I gave my mother a blank book with the instructions to write down any time God spoke to her in her heart. I just found this book last week and was struck by her December 13, 1976 entry:

"God spoke to me today and reminded me that there is one eternal truth which is love. Know that each person is a

child of God and deserves love. Bring to each person this spark of knowledge that God is with us and loves us. My special mission on earth is to love all people and to serve whenever needed. God who has been so good to me wants only that I show this love to others. I dedicate myself to this mission."

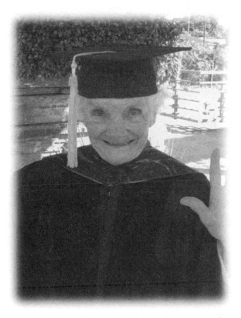

At her PhD graduation, Rami insisted her grandma try on the cap and gown. After she put it on and we took this photo, she said, "I want you to use this picture for my memorial so people will know I've graduated to my new life."

Well, Mom, I want to say to you that I am very proud of you for accomplishing your mission so perfectly. You deserve a PhD in Love and an MD for your healing power of love.

May we all now close our eyes for a moment and just feel her love for all of us in this church. Each one of us held a special place within her heart.

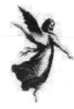

My mother's minister, Bob Bowles, led the service, and his love and devotion for my mom came through in every word he said. In typical fashion, my brother's talk was very funny as well as touching. Barry gave a beautiful talk and Rami read a very special poem she had written. (This poem is at the very end of the book.) Allen, my brother's son, played "Meditation by Thais" on his violin, which was breathtaking.

Then it came time for John-Nuri. Almost everyone who was attending the service had heard of Louise's request to her eighteen-year-old grandson to sing her Louise song. Everyone had also heard that she was "planning to sing along." John-Nuri sang her song so beautifully that there was not a dry eye in the church.

Grandma's Louise Song, as song by John-Nuri and Louise at her memorial service:

Every little breeze seems to whisper Louise
Birds in the trees seem to whisper Louise
Can it be true? Someone like you could love me, Louise.

Just to see and hear you
Is a joy I never knew
But to be so near you
Thrills me through and through.

Every little breeze seems to whisper Louise
Birds in the trees seem to whisper Louise
Can it be true? Someone like you could love me, Louise.

My mother lived a very simple life. She did not have a lot of money. There is no college building named in her honor, she was not a college professor, she never became famous (except to those whose lives were touched by her love), she never invented something, never came up with an idea that changed the world. Though it wasn't an original idea, she gave love, and that is what changes the world. Because of that love, which she generously gave to others, she touched the hearts of so many people. To me, that is a life well lived.

The reception after the memorial service was not a sad occasion. As a matter of fact, we all felt high on all the love. We were all feeling her caring for us over the years and that quality of unconditional love that she freely expressed. I believe we all knew that her love was a permanent part of us.

Conclusion

IN THE WEEKS FOLLOWING MY MOTHER'S DEATH, I realized I could now concentrate on enjoying her wisdom and love, without the time-consuming effort of caring for her worn-out old body. I started each day feeling her love for me and remembering her promise to never leave me. She also kept promising that when she passed from this world, she would again be able to care for me as a loving mother would. More and more I felt her loving care.

Five Christmases before she passed from this world, my mother gave me a small porcelain music box in the shape of a gift-wrapped box. When you open the lid, it plays the song, "Always." The inscription inside the lid reads, "Always my daughter, and now also my friend." A small hand-written note, also inside the box, brings me deep comfort: "Always remember, when you can no longer see me, I will still be there loving and caring for you. Your ever-loving Mom."

Because my mother lived her life with so much attention on love, I have wanted to emulate her, integrating some of her endearing qualities into my own life. She has taught me to be more grateful and take more opportunities to pray. She has taught me to be more expressive of love – not just with friends and family, but with people I don't know. I'm taking more time to stop and talk with people, rather than rushing by.

After a river trip last summer, Barry and I stopped at a little melon stand on the side of the road in Green River, Utah. After purchasing a few melons from an older couple, Barry saw that he needed a few things for our return trip and headed across the street to a hardware store. My usual mode of operation would have been to retreat into our camper and read. As I was heading for the camper, I thought about my mom and how she would have loved this opportunity to make new friends. When Barry returned from shopping, he found me selling a watermelon to a new customer and laughing with my two new friends. When Barry said it was time to go, I really didn't want to leave. As we were driving away, I felt an inner joy and could almost hear my mother saying, "Isn't it fun to make new friends!" As I bring my mother's strengths into my life, I feel closer to her and happier within myself.

I feel very grateful that I gave my mother so much of my time and energy in the last years, especially the last year of her life. I was able to comply with all of her wishes concerning her death. I am so grateful that we kept her at home, in a place where she felt so safe and secure. Our whole family knows that we gave her our all. Because of this, we had no regrets, which can be so burdensome after a person dies. In return, my mother gave us the valuable gift of being able to witness her dying process, which blessed all of our lives immensely. Her Hospice nurse, Carol, wrote after her passing, "Never lose sight of the great gift you all gave to your mother, and to yourselves, by letting her die in her own home."

My mother's death has changed my life. I've never been afraid of death itself. Rather, I've been afraid of the process it takes to get there. My mother's dying process played out my worst nightmare. She was incontinent, and had to have her granddaughters, daughter and son-in-law change messy, smelly diapers. She was totally dependent on other people for everything. She was not able to get a drink of water, go to the bathroom, or even change to a more comfortable position in bed. Plus, she was at times in tremendous pain.

I believe my mother concentrated on the goal rather than the inconveniences along the way. She had prepared her whole life for what she called, "the great adventure of death." The fact that this adventure had inconveniences, like being incontinent and in pain, did not stop her from enjoying the experience fully.

Imagine you had saved for many years to take a trip of a lifetime. You got to the airport and they told you your plane would be delayed. You might grumble a bit, but then just as quickly you would return to the excitement you felt about this dream trip. That's how my mother was. She grumbled a bit from time to time about the inconveniences of a failing body, but she held high the goal of a beautiful dying process -- a journey as well as a destination. There was so much about her dying experience that was exciting for her, like seeing my dad so clearly after eight years. That in itself was enough to erase anything painful or disturbing about the ordeal of dying. And that was just one thing. There was also seeing her mother after eighty-four years. And all of the spiritual experiences she was having of heavenly music, angels, visions and feeling the love of God so strongly around her. She never felt alone or scared. There was so much unseen help and love surrounding her.

Words from a song written by Michael Stillwater seem appropriate to what my mother was doing:

"Breathe in the pain, breathe on out the love. May my heart be a place where this world is changed forever."

I saw my mother doing this with her dying process. She was at times in tremendous pain and she breathed it in, then it went through her loving heart and she breathed out more love. In this way she showed me that it does not matter how our body dies. It matters that we concentrate on love and knowing we are being cared for in the highest way. Her main message to me on her death bed was, "Please tell everyone you can that death is *so* beautiful." My mother has given me many gifts in my life, but the model of dying in such a beautiful and grateful way was her final gift to me, and a gift I will greatly treasure. I can no longer be afraid of dying. No matter how difficult or complicated my own dying process becomes, her strength and positive attitude are now a part of me. I hope her messages have come through this book and touched your heart as well.

Our children are now thirty-two, twenty-six and nineteen as of this writing in 2008. I plan on sitting down with each one privately and saying, "When it is my time to die, I want you to be excited for me." I believe my dear mother will help me with these talks.

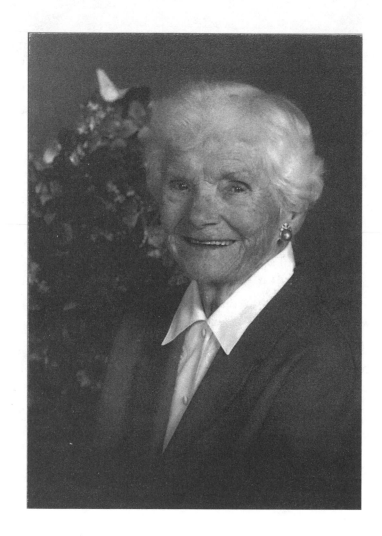

VISSELL

The Gift – by Rami Vissell

September 8, 2007

How do I capture the gift of death in words?
How do I convey the mystery unraveled,
The blessings illuminated?
Sleepless nights, I lay witness to heavenly dialogues
Well, one side of them anyway.
Countless gentle unseen beings fluttering in, fading
out.
The veil between worlds thin, at times blurred, at times
nonexistent.
I reached out to touch you,
Wishing to take the pain away from you.
Your body ebbing, yet glorious.
And you reached out to touch me,
Beyond where sensation can go.
You showed me in timeless moments a place so heaven-
ly, so gracious, so vast…
That death's shadow was no more than a bell
Marking the beginning of an incredible journey.
And why not rejoice in this beginning?
I feel so lucky to come along with you for your first few
steps.

Tears? Yes.
Joy? Yes!
Death, birth, you taught me that life certainly goes on.
What a gift you gave me,
To deeply know of the peace that awaits me, and all of
us, beyond these bodies.
No fear is necessary, just a gentle exhale, and away we
go, free!
I am so honored.
Thank you, Grandma.
I love you!

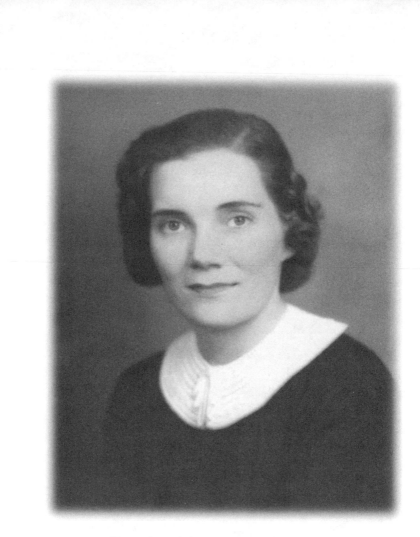

Even though Louise was only twenty in
this photo, this was the expression on her
face as she took her final breaths.

WE HOPE YOU HAVE ENJOYED READING this important message from Louise. We'd like to ask for your help to make her message available to others.

A Mother's Final Gift is not published by a major publishing house with a big marketing budget. It is published by our family. We do not have a marketing budget, but are having faith that people will help us to get this message and inspiration out to others.

If everyone who reads this could recommend it to a few people, it would help us enormously. It can be ordered on Amazon.com (paper or download), as well as our website (SharedHeart.org), or from calling us at Ramira Publishing (800.766.0629).

Another option is listening to this book, recorded by each member of our family in their own voices (audio CD's or downloaded for playing on your digital audio device).

We so appreciate your help and support. May Louise and her band of angels bless your life. Thank you.

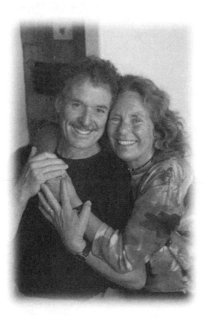

Joyce and Barry Vissell are best known as relationship experts who have helped many thousands of people through their books, workshops and counseling practice since 1975. They have found that the power of love can heal even the most troubled relationships.

They are two people deeply in love for 46 years, who have raised three children and "walk their talk." As a result of the interest in their books, *The Shared Heart, Models of Love, Risk To Be Healed, Light in the Mirror,* and *Meant To Be,* they have been conducting talks and workshops on relationship and personal growth world-wide. They are the founders and directors of the Shared Heart Foundation, a non-profit organization dedicated to changing the world one heart at a time. Joyce and Barry live at their home and center with their three golden retrievers and one cat in the Santa Cruz Mountains of Central California.

Go to **SharedHeart.org** to sign up for their **free heartletter**, to read past articles on many aspects of personal growth and relationship, to see their event or workshop schedule, or to contact Barry or Joyce.

Rami Vissell has a PhD in Clinical Psychology and has a private practice working in person or by phone with teens and parents. She is the author of *Rami's Book: The inner life of a Child*. She lives in Aptos, CA, with her husband River and their son, Skye, born Jan 14, 2011.

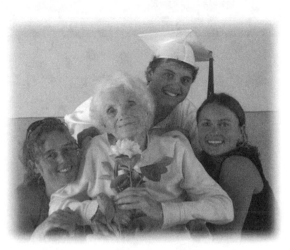

John-Nuri graduates from High School three months before Louise's passing. Rami is on the left, Mira on the right.

Mira Vissell received her BS from UC Santa Cruz. She has completed all the requirements for nursing school and is on the waiting list for the next available school. She is currently our part-time office assistant as well as care-giving and rehabilitating a disabled woman. She lives with her golden retriever, Maggie, in Santa Cruz.

John-Nuri will be graduating in May, 2011, from Lewis and Clark College in Portland, OR, with a degree in Psychology and Hispanic Studies. He loves to sing and is a member of the college choir. He is a licensed massage practitioner and volunteers for Hospice.

ALSO BY THE VISSELLS

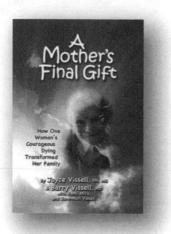

A MOTHER'S FINAL GIFT (RECORDED AUDIO BOOK)

Recorded by the Vissell family in their own voices, each member speaking (and sometimes singing) their own part. This inspiring audio book would be ideal while driving, or for family or group listening.

Available on CDs or download to your own audio player from SharedHeart.org.

**Available on SharedHeart.org or by calling toll-free
800.766.0629**

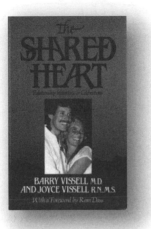

THE SHARED HEART

Relationship Initiations
and Celebrations

ISBN 0-9612720-0-7, 186 pages, ©1984, Ramira Publishing, $9.95

The Shared Heart was one of the first books to bridge the chasm between following a spiritual path and having a deeply committed love relationship. As the book says, "Loving one other person teaches you how to love all people."

"First the One became the many. Now the many are uniting back into the One by the miracle of love. Barry and Joyce, in The Shared Heart, show how the human relationship is the first step." **—Pir Vilayat Khan, former head of the Sufi Order of America**

"The Shared Heart is full of beauty and compassion, richness and clarity. Barry and Joyce plough through the hard and soft spaces of the journey with great inner strength and deep respect for reflective inner tuning." **—Ram Dass**

"From the perspectives of romance, marriage, making love, parenting, careers, spiritual initiation, and loss of a loved one, this remarkable couple exhibits insight, acceptance and transcendence, at the same time offering specific tools for the transformational process of love." **—Yoga Journal**

Available on SharedHeart.org or by calling toll-free
800.766.0629

MODELS OF LOVE
The Parent-Child Journey
ISBN 0-9612720-1-5, 320 pages, ©1986, Ramira
Publishing, $12.95

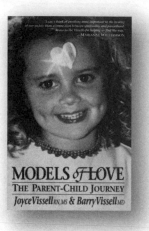

Contributors include Jack Kornfield, Eileen Caddy, Leo Buscaglia, Jerry Jampolsky, Joan Hodgson, Jeannine Parvati Baker and others.

"Our children need not fall asleep to the beauty of their heavenly state for twenty, thirty, or more years, at which time breaking the habit of material thought is very difficult. We can help them begin the awakening process from the day they are conceived, so that the bridge of consciousness between the two worlds is continually strengthened."

"This is a book we whole-heartedly recommend to first-time parents, to grandparents, and to everyone in between." —**Mothering Magazine**

"Models of Love is more than a parenting book. It will bless your whole life!" —**John Bradshaw**

"This book is full of miraculous incidents and sacred moments of loving connection that will bring tears to your eyes." —**Whole Life Magazine**

"What society needs most is a connection between spirituality and parenthood. Bravo to the Vissells for helping us find the way" —**Marianne Williamson.**

Available on SharedHeart.org or by calling toll-free 800.766.0629

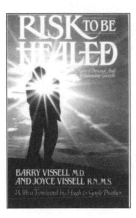

RISK TO BE HEALED
The Heart of Personal and Relationship Growth

ISBN 0-9612720-2-3, 192 pages, ©1989, Ramira Publishing, $9.95

Not infrequently, we receive an email or a letter with the words, "Your book has changed my life." Almost without exception, the writer is referring to *Risk to Be Healed*.

"In this book, Joyce & Barry offer the priceless gift of their own experience with relationship, commitment, vulnerability, and loss, along with the profound guide to healing that comes from the core of their being and blesses us with gentle wisdom." —**Gayle & Hugh Prather**

The Vissells, in their uniquely captivating and personally revealing way, extend another written offering to the world. *Risk to be Healed* is filled with stories from their own continuing growth, as well as the healing risks individuals and couples have taken in their counseling sessions and workshops. The book begins with the profound experience of Anjel's death in utero and her subsequent birth into the lives of the authors. Subject matter includes: risk-taking in relationship, the way of intimacy, the power of right livelihood, understanding pain, healing relationships with those who have passed on, addictions, appreciation, vulnerability, and simplifying our lives.

Available on SharedHeart.org or by calling toll-free 800.766.0629

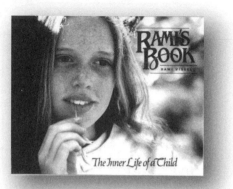

Rami's Book

The Inner Life of a Child

by Rami Vissell

ISBN 0-9612720-4-X, hardcover,
56 pages, full-color illustrated,
©1989, Ramira Publishing, $13.95

"We have been taught for a long time that the entrance to God's presence is through the eyes of a child. Rami flings wide that delicious door of perception." **—Rev. Stan Hampson, Past President, Association of Unity Churches**

"My hope is that all adults as well as children may benefit by the understanding and love that Rami shares in this delightful book." **—Ken Keyes**

"Rami's book is a gift from an angel. The innocent beauty filling these pages brings me tears of joy. I wish children of all ages would read this book." **—Alan Cohen**

"Sensitively and endearingly written ... Rami's innocence and candidness is both moving and refreshing." **—Science of Thought Review, England**

"Of all the books I've reviewed, this one went right to my heart and made me cry quite wonderfully. Truly an angelic and marvelous work, and a gift to the child still within me. I put it on display with a sign: 'very, very highly recommended. 4 stars on the goose bump chart!'." **—Richard Rodgers, manager, The Grateful Heart Bookstore.**

**Available on SharedHeart.org or by calling toll-free
800.766.0629**

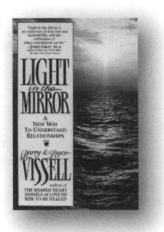

LIGHT IN THE MIRROR
A New Way to Understand Relationships
ISBN: 0-9612720-5-8, ©1995, Ramira Publishing, $13.95

"Light in the Mirror *is an expression of deep love and vulnerability, and the celebration of what commitment can be." —* **John Gray, PhD**, author of *Men Are From Mars, Women Are From Venus.*

"*In* Light in the Mirror, *Joyce and Barry Vissell share with deep tenderness and vulnerability the valleys and peaks of their relationship. They go on to share 'practical spirituality,' suggestions that will be most helpful to everyone finding their way home to the heart." —* **Gerald Jampolsky, MD** and **Diane Cirincione**, authors of *Love is the Answer* and *Change Your Mind, Change Your Life.*

"*We have always benefited from the gentle wisdom of the Vissells.* Light in the Mirror *is one of the rare voices for sanity in the field of relationships." —* **Gayle and Hugh Prather**, authors of *Notes to Myself* and *I Will Never Leave You.*

"*If you had but one book to choose to renew your relationship, this should be the one." —***Small Press Magazine**

"*Light in the Mirror is a must for anyone who yearns for better connection and more joy in their intimate relationships." —***Napra Review**

Available on SharedHeart.org or by calling toll-free 800.766.0629

MEANT TO BE

Miraculous True Stories To Inspire A Lifetime Of Love

ISBN 1-57324-161-X, ©2000, Conari Press, $14.95

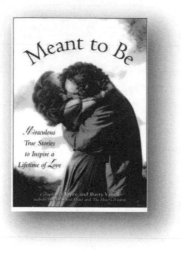

"The true miracle of these stories is that they open your heart to your own miracle, for the miracle of love is within you too, and your story can be as magical as these. That is the healing message on Meant to Be, that is its wonder." – **Neale Donald Walsch**, author of *Conversations with God*

"Few books make me cry, but this one did, many times. The best collection of heart-full stories that I have ever read!" – **Mary Jane Ryan**, author of *Random Acts of Kindness*

"These wonderful stories remind us of the miracle that love is, and the magical ways it comes into our lives. Meant To Be *proves that, at the deepest levels, destiny is always at work in our lives."* —**Susannah Seton, author of Simple Pleasures**

Available on SharedHeart.org or by calling toll-free 800.766.0629